ESSENTIAL FATTY ACIDS
AND INFANT NUTRITION

British Library Cataloguing in Publication Data
A catalogue record for this book is available from the British Library.

ISBN 0 86196 395-4

Editions John Libbey Eurotext
6, rue Blanche, 92120 Montrouge, France. Tél.: (1) 47.35.85.52

John Libbey & Company Ltd
13, Smith Yard, Summerley Street, London SW18 4HR, England
Tel.: (01) 947.27.77

John Libbey CIC
Via L. Spallanzani, 11, 00161 Rome, Italy. Tel.: (06) 862.289

© John Libbey Eurotext, 1992, Paris

Il est interdit de reproduire intégralement ou partiellement le présent ouvrage - loi du 11 mars 1957 - sans autorisation de l'éditeur ou du Centre Français du Copyright, 6 *bis*, rue Gabriel Laumain, 75010 Paris

ESSENTIAL FATTY ACIDS AND INFANT NUTRITION

Proceedings of the International Symposium
May 26-27, 1989, Athens, Greece

Edited by
J. Ghisolfi
G. Putet

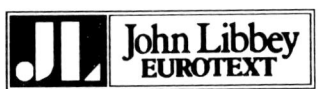   *milupa*

Foreword

Milupa has a long standing reputation for conducting detailed foundation research into the nature of human breastmilk. Key areas of interest include fats, proteins, and carbohydrates. This work has provided the basis for the development of a number of standard infant formulas and special products for particular nutritional needs.

On the other hand the success of many development projects was only possible with the co-operation of clinicians at hospitals all over Europe. Milupa recognize that if they are to stay in the forefront of the infant nutrition market, this commitment to research needs to continue. This symposium, consequently, represents one example of how mutualistic exchange of views and clinical practice can result in defining the direction of future research and development. Although predominantly active in Europe Milupa did not hesitate to ask renowned experts from all over the world (including the USA and Canada) to participate in this meeting as to generate a most complete "state of the art" in the area of Essential Fatty Acids and Infant Nutrition.

Thanks to the excellent preparation of this meeting by the scientific organizers, Prof J. Ghisolfi and Dr G. Putet, and thanks to the very interesting presentations of all speakers and the stimulating discussions among all experts this symposium was a success. We would like to express our gratitude to all of them.

G. Olesch

List of participants

Béréziat G., Laboratoire de Biochimie, URA CNRS 1283, Faculté de Médecine Saint-Antoine, 27, rue Chaligny, 75571 Paris Cedex 12, France.

Bitman J., Milk Secretion and Mastitis Laboratory, USDA-ARS, Beltsville, MD, USA.

Boulot P., Département d'Obstétrique, CHU Lapeyronie, 34060 Montpellier Cedex, France.

Bourre J.M., INSERM U. 26, Hôpital Fernand-Widal, 200, rue du Faubourg Saint-Denis, 75475 Paris Cedex 10, France.

Cardot P., Département de Nutrition Humaine, INRA-Theix, Clermond-Ferrand, France.

Carlson S.E., College of Medicine, Department of Pediatrics, 853 Jefferson Avenue, Memphis, TN 38163, USA.

Chambaz J., Laboratoire de Biochimie, URA CNRS 1283, Faculté de Médecine Saint-Antoine, 27, rue Chaligny, 75571 Paris Cedex 12, France.

Chirouze V., IMEDEX, Z.I. des Troques, BP 38, 69630 Chaponost, France.

Clandinin M.T., University of Alberta, Faculty of Medicine, Nutrition and Metabolism Research Group, 533 Newton Research Building, Edmonton, Alberta, Canada.

Cooke R.J., College of Medicine, Department of Pediatrics, 853 Jefferson Avenue, Memphis, TN 38163, USA.

Crastes de Paulet A., Laboratoire de Biochimie A, CHU Lapeyronie, 34060 Montpellier Cedex, France.

Crastes de Paulet P., Laboratoire de Biochimie A, CHU Lapeyronie, 34060 Montpellier Cedex, France.

Debray J., Milupa, «Les Mercuriales», 40, rue Jean-Jaurès, 93176 Bagnolet Cedex, France.

Dupuy R.P., Hôpital Saint-Charles, Service de Pédiatrie Néonatale, CHRU de Montpellier, 34059 Montpellier Cedex, France.

Galli C., Universita di Milano, Instituto di Scienze Farmacologiche, Cattedra Di Saggi E, Via Balzaretti, 9, 20133 Milano, Italy.

Ghisolfi J., Service de Médecine Infantile D, CHU Purpan, Hôpital de Purpan, Place du Docteur-Baylac, 31059 Toulouse Cedex, France.

Hamosh M., Department of Pediatrics, Georgetown University Children's Medical Center, 3800 Reservoir Road NW, Washington DC 20007-2197, USA.

Hernell O., Department of Physiological Chemistry, University of Umea, 90185 Umea, Sweden.

Hull D., Department of Child Health, Floor E, East Block, University Hospital, Queen's Medical Center, Nottingham NG7 2 UH, England, United Kingdom.

Inacio J., Milupa, «Les Mercuriales», 40, rue Jean-Jaurès, 93176 Bagnolet Cedex, France.

Innis S., University of British Columbia, B.C. Children's Hospital, Research Center, Shaughnessy Site, 950 - West 28th Avenue, Vancouver, British Columbia, Canada V5Z4HA, Canada.

Iverson S.J., Department of Pediatrics, Georgetown University Children's Medical Center, 3800 Reservoir Road NW, Washington DC 20007-2197, USA.

Kohn G., Milupa AG, Bahnstrasse, D-6382 Friedrichsdorf/Ts, Germany.

Koletzko B., Kinderklinik der Heinrich-heine-Universität, Moorenstr. 5, D-4000 Düsseldorf 1, Germany.

Mehta N.R., Department of Pediatrics, Georgetown University Children's Medical Center, 3800 Reservoir Road NW, Washington DC 20007-2197, USA.

Olesch G., Milupa AG, Bahnstrasse, D-6382 Friedrichsdorf/Ts, Germany.

Peeples J.M., College of Medicine, Department of Pediatrics, 853 Jefferson Avenue, Memphis, TN 38163, USA.

Pita M.L., Universidad de Granada, Departamento de Bioquimica y Biologica Molecular, Facultad de Ciencias, 18071 Granada, Spain.

Putet G., Service de Néonatologie et de Réanimation Néonatale, Hôpital Debrousse, 69322 Lyon Cedex 05, France.

Ramet J.L., Milupa, «Les Mercuriales», 40, rue Jean-Jaurès, 93176 Bagnolet Cedex, France.

Rey J., Département de Pédiatrie, Hôpital Necker-Enfants Malades, 149, rue de Sèvres, 75743 Paris Cedex 15, France.

Rieu D., Clinique des Enfants Malades, Hôpital Saint-Charles, 300, rue Auguste-Broussonet, 34059 Montpellier Cedex, France.

Rigo J., Service Universitaire de Néonatologie, Hôpital de la Citadelle, Boulevard du 12e de ligne 1, 4000 Belgium.

Salle B., Service de Néonatologie et de Réanimation Néonatale, Hôpital Edouard-Herriot, Place d'Arsonval, 69437 Lyon Cedex 03, France.

Sarda P., Service de Néonatologie, CHU Lapeyronie, 34060 Montpellier Cedex, France.

Sawatzki G., Milupa AG, Bahnstrasse, D-6382 Friedrichsdorf/Ts Germany.

Spear M.L., Division of Neonatalogy, Medical Center of Delaware and E. Jefferson Medical College, Philadelphia, PA, USA.

Thomas G., Laboratoire de Biochimie, URA CNRS 1283, Faculté de Médecine Saint-Antoine, 27, rue Chaligny, 75571 Paris Cedex 12, France.

Tolley E.A., College of Medicine, Department of Pediatrics, 853 Jefferson Avenue, Memphis, TN 38163, USA.

Van Aerde J., University of Alberta, Faculty of Medicine, Nutrition and Metabolism Research Group, 533 Newton Research Building, Edmonton, Alberta, Canada.

Vidailhet M., Service de Médecine Infantile "3", CHRU de Nancy, Hôpitaux de Brabois, rue du Morvan, 54511 Vandœuvre Cedex, France.

Werkman S.H., College of Medicine, Department of Pediatrics, 853 Jefferson Avenue, Memphis, TN 38163, USA.

Contents

Foreword (G. Olesch, Germany) V
List of participants VII
Introductory remarks. J. Ghisolfi (France), G. Putet (France), J. Rey (France). XIII
Preface. J. Rey (France) XV

Session I. Chairman: A. Crastes de Paulet (France)

1. Membranes and essential fatty acids (except the neural system). G. Galli (Italy) 3
2. Essential fatty acids and brain development and function. J.M. Bourre (France) 11
3. Essential fatty acid composition of tissue lipids in the perinatal period. M.T. Clandinin, J. Van Aerde (Canada) 23

Session II. Chairman: S. Carlson (USA)

4. Effects of current infant formula on brain and retinal lipid development. Effect of formula with 2% 18:3 n-3 on n-6 and n-3 fatty acid status of low birthweight infants. S. Innis (Canada) 31
5. Essential fatty acid interconversion during the perinatal period. Influence of dietary factors. G. Béréziat, G. Thomas, P. Cardot, J. Chambaz (France) 45

Session III. Chairman: D. Hull (United Kingdom)

6. Role of the placenta in the foetus fatty acids supply. V. Chirouze (France) 59

7. Fatty acids blood composition in foetal and maternal plasma. P. Crastes de Paulet, P. Sarda, P. Boulot, A. Crastes de Paulet (France)   65
8. Human milk and fatty acids: quantitative aspects. G. Kohn (Germany)   79

Session IV. Chairman: S. Innis (Canada)

9. Human milk and fatty acids: qualitative aspects. P. Sarda, D. Rieu (France)   91
10. Human milk nucleotides and essential fatty acid metabolism during early life. M.L. Pita (Spain)   101

Session V. Chairman: J.M. Bourre (France)

11. Docosahexaenoate (DHA) and eicosapentaenoate (EPA) supplementation of preterm (PT) infants: effects on RBC and plasma N-3 and visual acuity. S.E. Carlson, R.J. Cooke, J.M. Peeples, S.H. Werkman, E.A. Tolley (USA)   111
12. Lipids in human milk and their digestion by the newborn infant. M. Hamosh, S.J. Iverson, N.R. Mehta, M.L. Spear, J. Bitman (USA)   119

Session VI. Round table. Chairman: J. Rey (France)

13. How to appreciate an inadequate essential fatty acid intake in infancy. J. Ghisolfi (France)   141
14. Minimal, optimal, maximal essential fatty acid requirements during infancy: term infants. B. Koletzko (Germany)   147
15. Essential fatty acid requirements in premature infants. G. Putet (France)   157
16. Omega-3 and omega-6 fatty acid supplementation in infant formulas. G. Sawatzki (Germany)   165

Session VII. General discussion. Chairman: J. Rey (France)   175

Introductory remarks

Ladies and gentlemen,

You are very welcome to this workshop on Essential Fatty Acids and Infant Nutrition.

Some thousand years ago, when man learnt to domesticate animals, non human milk became available to supplement or replace the mother's milk. By replacing human milk with cow's milk and secondary industrial formulas, a new challenge was imposed on medical professionals: the nutritional requirements of the infant had to be determined. One of these requirements concerns essential fatty acids.

It is no longer debated that fatty acid supplies by milks are very important for infant development. In order to correct the dissimilarities in fatty acid composition between human milk and cow milk, manufacturers replaced part of the bovine milk fat with vegetable oils. These progressive changes of the fat supplement led to a fatty acid profile in formulas better adapted to infant needs. We are however very far from fatty acid composition of human milk and a lot of questions remain to be debated to improve the nutritional qualities of infant formulas.

Now, the rapid increase in our knowledge on fatty acids in infant nutrition has created the need for a critical appraisal of the state of the art. So, we thought, it was time to arrange a symposium with the very best specialists in the field of essential fatty acids and infant nutrition, to obtain a proper picture on this topic.

When we spoke of this idea to Mr Olesch and Mr Ramet from Milupa France, they immediately proposed to help us in the organisation of this meeting. As you know, Milupa France entirely sponsored it. If we are lucky to be here, in Greece, it is on suggestion of Mr Olesch and Mr Ramet. Many thanks to them. Without their constant help, perhaps the meeting would not be taking place.

We are proud and happy to have managed to get those who are recognized as being the best on this topic. Thank you very much to everybody.

Let us now turn to the topics of the symposium:
– this morning, we will speak about basis knowledge on linoleic alphalinolenic and polyunsaturated fatty acid metabolism during the growing period;
– in the afternoon, we will consider the fatty acid supplies during pregnancy and after birth. We will particularly look at the human milk composition;
– tomorrow morning, we will begin by considerations about long chain polyunsaturated fatty acids and infant nutrition and the consequences of an inadequate essential fatty acid intake in infancy. We will finish our symposium by a round table which might allow us to exchange our ideas on the better fatty acid composition of infant formulas.

We have much to learn about essential fatty acids and infant nutrition. We hope that at the end of this workshop we shall have a better understanding of the problem posed.

J. Ghisolfi
G. Putet
J. Rey

Preface

J. REY
Département de Pédiatrie, Hôpital Necker Enfants-Malades,
149, rue de Sèvres, 75743 Paris Cedex 15, France

The interest of scientists and manufacturers in essential fatty acids is not new. Sixty years ago Burr and Burr gave evidence of linoleic acid as an essential constituent of fat [1] and just about 30 years ago Hansen *et al.* reported in two famous supplements of *Acta Paediatrica* and *Pediatrics* on the results of studies investigating the importance of linoleic acid in infant nutrition [2, 3]. The essential role of fatty acids of the n-3 (or omega-3) series for a long time considered as secondary was confirmed on the other hand during the past 15 years. Today everyone agrees that α–linolenic acid and its long chain derivatives, particularly docosahexaenoic acid (DHA), are essential components of brain and retina and are of crucial importance for the development of these organs. Further they are known for their hypolipidaemic and antithrombotic effects, their immunologic and anticancerogenic actions and their possible effect on the duration of gestation [4, 5].

Consequently, a lot of problems are actually solved. However, some problems deserve all our attention. The type of fat and the relative proportions of different essential and non-essential fatty acid families as part of the alimentation have an influence on the structure and fluidity of membranes and thus on a certain number of functions, especially, if diet-induced modifications affect the central nervous system at the moment of its biochemical and functional maturation [6]. In this respect, studies investigating the effects in premature infants fed formulas supplemented with long chain polyunsaturated fatty acids, e.g. effects such as the phospholipid composition of erythrocytes [7], visual acuity and evoked potentials [8], are of prime importance for future recommendations [9]. This also means a challenge for manufacturers because of the difficulties to prepare mixtures the composition of which comes closer every day to that of human milk and due to the fact that polyunsaturated fatty acids are highly susceptible to oxidation.

In this regard, it is gratifying to see that scientists, clinicians and manufacturers meet together to discuss and exchange their points of view. It is by way of these confrontations that ideas are brought forth and that the different groups come to a better understanding of each other and clear away any distrust. Consequently, we feel grateful to Jacques Ghisolfi, Guy Putet and Milupa for the organisation of this conference the content of which is published in this book.

References

1. Burr G.O., Burr M.M. A new deficiency disease produced by the rigid exclusion of fat from the diet. *J Biol Chem* 1930; 86:587.
2. Hansen A.E., Stewart R.A., Hugues G., Soderhjelm L. The relation of linoleic acid to infant feeding. A review. *Acta Paediatrica* 1962; 51, suppl. 137.

3. Hansen A.E., Wiese H.F., Boelsche A.N. *et al.* Role of linoleic acid in infant nutrition. *Pediatrics* 1963; 31: N° 1, part II (suppl).
4. Neuringer M., Anderson G.L., Connor W.E. The essentiality of n-3 fatty acids for the development and function of the retina and brain. *Annu Rev Nutr* 1988; 8:517-41
5. Nestel P.J. Effects of n-3 fatty acids on lipid metabolism. *Annu Rev Nutr* 1990; 10:149-67.
6. Innis S.M. Lipids in infant nutrition. Introduction. *J Pediatr* 1992; 120, n° 4, part 2 (suppl).
7. Carlson S.E., Cooke R.J., Rhodes P.G. *et al.* Long term feeding of formulas high in linolenic acid and marine oil to very low birth weight infants: phospholipid fatty acids. *Pediatr Res* 1991; 30:404-12.
8. Uauy R., Birch E., Birch D., Peirano P. Visual and brain function measurements in studies of n-3 fatty acid requirements of infants. *J Pediatr* 1992; 120:168-80.
9. ESPGAN Committee on Nutrition. Comment on the content and composition of lipids in infant formulas. *Acta Paediatr Scand* 1991; 80:887-96.

SESSION I

Chairman: A. CRASTES DE PAULET (France)

1

Membranes and essential fatty acids (except the neural system)

C. GALLI

Universita di Milano, Instituto di Scienze Farmacologiche, Cattedra Di Saggi E, Via Balzcretti, 9, 20133 Milano, Italy

First of all I wish to address my gratitude to the organisers, specially Prof Ghisolfi and Dr Putet for giving me the opportunity to come to this interesting meeting on EFA in Infant Nutrition in the city of Athens. I feel it's quite appropriate to have a meeting on a topic which requires a lot of wisdom in a city which has got the name of the Goddess of Wisdom.

Some lipids have attracted the attention of biochemists and people working with the biological membranes for several years, but only recently has the interest into cell lipids been extended also to cell biologists, pharmacologists, physiologists due to the increasing evidence for a role of cell lipids in the regulation of several cell functions.

Recent studies on the metabolism of dietary fatty acids have given a considerable contribution to this knowledge both from a quantitative and qualitative point of view.

In the current view, integral membrane proteins are strictly associated with inner phospholipids; on the exterior face of the membrane the carbohydrate chains of the glycoproteins and glycolipids are extended into the medium.

The lipid patches of different composition aggregate and they segregate to form separate lipid domains. The type of fatty acids which are included in the complex lipid components may contribute to modulate the properties of the domain. This cytosolic face of the membrane has an extensive lipid surface, including various components. The whole thing is a dynamic structure and each class of components undergoes different varieties of motion on different time scales.

Several properties of the lipid phase in the membrane can be quantified. Lipid dynamics is frequently referred to as membrane fluidity, a term which refers to the physical state and structure of the fatty acid chains comprising the membrane structure. The "chain order", a term which implies a restriction on mobility, increases with increasing chain length of the fatty acids, but also with decreasing unsaturation. Also the correlations between fluidity, phase transition temperature and desaturation indexes, which are frequently given in literature, are rather complex. Not only the number of double bonds but also the position of double bonds is very critical, especially position of the initial double bond in the molecule. Lipid asymmetry has been described for several types of cells in addition to asymmetric distribution of phospholipids and cholesterol across the membrane; also the fatty acids might be asymmetrically distributed, not only as a consequence of the characteristic distribution of fatty acids and molecular phospholipid classes, but also because of different fatty acid profiles in the same phospholipid in the different sides of the membrane. It has been shown that fatty acid profiles in the exterior and interior face of the synaptic membranes, in the same phospholipid, have a different content of unsaturated fatty acid. The different fatty acid composition on the two sides of the membrane raises the possibility that membrane enzymes could be modulated differently too by this difference. Lateral domains may arise from fluid fluid as well as fluid solid miscibility and these may be seen as distinct lipid structures. Large scale domains have been studied in detail in the liver cells [1] which can be dissected in three different regions, the blood sinusoidal, the contiguous and the bile canalicular leaflets. For instance, the proportion of PE which is placed exofacially in the sinusoidal and the bile canicular segment is much higher than in the other section. So even if the total amount of PEs is the same in all the different types of membranes, there is a different distribution within the membrane and the same phospholipid. And it is of interest that each region has a distinct set of functions. Adenylatecyclase for instance is mainly located in the blood sinusoidal whereas the ATPase is mainly located in the contiguous fraction. So the different distribution of phospholipids, in different domains, may be associated with different functions.

In addition to the well known and long studied role of phospholipids, in the modulation of some physico-chemical parameters in the membrane, membrane lipids are also involved in the modulation of several functional aspects of cells through the formation of different metabolites. All these processes are triggered by activation of phospholipases, enzymes which break down specific phospholipids, releasing biologically active products. Different phospholipases are recognized depending upon the site of action of the phospholipid molecule. Among the products which are generated and which are known to be very active in several biological systems, the eicosanoids are derived directly from the polyunsaturated fatty acid arachidonic acid, which is released through various pathways. The compound platelet activity factor (PAF) is also produced after activation of phospholipase A2 acting on a phosphatidylcholine containing another function in position 1 of glycerol, followed by acetylation in position 2. Both eicosanoid and PAF are very important compounds mediating intercellular responses in various types of cells. On the other side the products derived from the activation of phospholipase C acting on phosphoinositides, giving life to the glycerol and inosotol phosphate are important mediators in the activation of intracellular events. Thus, the modulation of polyunsaturated fatty acids in cell membranes can either directly affect the eicosanoid pathway, by changing the proportion in the levels of the polyunsaturated fatty acid precursors or also indirectly may affect some of the pathways, for the synthesis of lipid mediators, through modification of the activity of the enzymes which are involved in the synthesis.

An important point concerning the fatty acids in tissue lipids is that each phospholipid class in membranes has a characteristic fatty acid profile. It appears, thus, that various mechanisms are operating in the control of fatty acid group composition of membranes. To some extent, however, the changes in the absolute levels and in the proportion of fatty acids in the diet may modulate the fatty acid composition of cell lipids. Some of the factors involved in the control of membrane fatty acids have been studied. Interactions occuring in the endoplasmic reticulum, mainly in the hepatocytes, at least in the adult organism are desaturation and elongation reactions of fatty acids. In addition phospholipid synthesis and exchange processes may contribute to modulate the fatty acid profile. Other reactions affecting membrane fatty acids occur during the process of membrane assembly. Finally, within the membrane fatty acid, modifications directly on the phospholipid molecules can take place through phospholipase action, acylation, transacylation and exchange of head groups.

An important aspect in the overall utilization of EFAs in various organs and tissues is represented by the relationships between the liver and extrahepatic tissues. Metabolism of linoleic and alphalinolenic acid occur mainly in the liver, whereas in extra hepatic tissues, many other processes, which have been previously mentioned, are operating. These processes regulate utilization of polyunsaturated acids by cells: acylco As specific for different fatty acids have been recognized in different tissues, specific reactions for arachidonic acid or 22:6, being very active, for instance, in the heart. The incorporation into specific phospholipids desaturation, elongation and retroconversion reactions are additional processes occuring in extra-hepatic tissues. Desaturation and elongation of fatty acids have been studied in great detail, especially in the liver, and it appears that competition between different substrates influences the pathways for the synthesis or the conversion of different polyunsaturates. So that the well known accumulation in tissues of eicosatrienoic fatty acid, derived from oleic acid, which is recognized as a marker of essential fatty acid deficiency, is mainly due to a release of the inhibition of the desaturation and elongation of oleic acid to this fatty acid. The role of the liver in supplying polyunsaturated fatty acid to peripheral tissues is illustrated by several studies. In one of these studies we carried out years ago [2], we observed that during essential fatty acid deficiency, induced in the label from birth, the total levels of polyunsaturated fatty acids, such as arachidonic acid, vary in a different way in the brain and in the liver. In fact, under these conditions there is a marked depletion of arachidonic acid in the liver, whereas at the same time arachidonic acid accumulates in the brain. With regards to the fatty acids, liver and platelets represent, two extreme types of cells, one having a good capacity for desaturation and elongation of fatty acids, whereas in the other the replacement of fatty acid in phospholipid is the major process. We could see that as a consequence of high linoleic acid, there was an elevation of both linoleic and arachidonic acids in the liver, whereas in platelets there was a replacement of arachidonic acid by the excess linoleic acid. As a consequence, we could see that after supplying high linoleic with the diet, the unsaturation index (an index, which can be easily calculated by multiplying the percentage of each fatty acid by the number of double bonds, and adding up the values), which is an indication on the total number of double bonds of each fatty acid, was increased in the liver, because the total polyunsaturates increased. On the other side the arachidonic/linoleic acid ratio remained constant because more linoleic acid enters the liver, more arachidonic acid is produced. The desaturation index in liver phospholipid is, thus, quite high when we feed high linoleic acid. In platelets, and in other cells, when we give high linoleic acid in the diet, the arachidonic acid/linoleic acid ratio in contrast with the situation in the liver is changed, in respect to values in a situation of low dietary linoleic acid. With high dietary linoleic acid, the arachidonic/linoleic acid ratio in platelet phospholipids is lower than in the condition of low dietary linoleic acid. This is due to the lack of desaturation of linoleic acid in platelets and to replacement of arachidonic acid by linoleic acid. There are, thus, different types of modification of cell fatty acids in different tissues, after high dietary linoleic acid: elongation and desaturation vs replacement.

The influence of dietary fatty acids on cell and tissue functions can be assessed by increasing changes of different biological parameters. Essential fatty acid deficiency, for instance, can affect the activity of various types of membranes of several enzymes. The activity of the enzymes involved in phospholipid synthesis is increased, the coupling of oxidation is reduced, the utilization of glucose by oxidating pathways is reduced; other processes are also affected.

Some enzymes have been studied more in detail, especially the sodium potassium ATPase in various organs including the liver. These enzymes are lipid requiring enzymes, because they need a lipid micro-environment in order to operate properly. There are several studies [5] indicating that by changing the composition of the diet, especially by inducing EFA deficiency, the activity of these enzymes is dramatically affected. In the liver, during EFA deficiency, the adenylatecyclase activity is decreased, and also, the response of the ATPase to different stimulating compounds is affected by the type of diet which is given to animals.

Also the influences of essential fatty acids on different parameters, including functional parameters, have been studied in *in vitro* systems, and the results indicate that essential fatty acid supplementation modifies different functions in different cells. Lymphocyte transformation is increased in low concentration and depressed in high concentration of the essential fatty acids in the medium. Cell fusion is enhanced. However these studies were carried out in *in vitro* systems and it may be difficult to extrapolate the results to the *in vivo* situation. Of course, the most predictable biological effects are those related to changes of levels of the precursors of eicosanoids due to manipulations of the diet. Thus, EFA deficiency depresses the accumulation of arachidonic and also of eicosapentaenoic acid in the tissues, so that the production of eicosanoids derived from these 20 carbon polyunsaturates is depressed. Also, the accumulation of trienoic becomes completely depleted of arachidonic acid, then eicosatrienoic acid begins to accumulate in the brain. This suggests that the liver is supplying polyunsaturated fatty acid to the brain. When arachidonic acid stores in the liver are completely depleted, then brain starts taking up the other polyunsaturated fatty acids, such as eicosatrienoic acid. Similarly, it has been shown by the group of Needleman [3] more recently that during essential fatty deficiency, the injection of arachidonate gives rise to a rapid incorporation of the label in the liver and this is followed later on by accumulation in tissues such as the heart and the kidney. There are also different responses of tissues to essential fatty acid deficiency and this can be seen by comparing the trienoic/tetraenoic ratio, which is the biochemical marker of EFA deficiency, in various phospholipids in different tissues. During essential fatty acid deficiency in mice, this ratio is generally higher in liver and in kidney medulla than in the heart and in the renal cortex. Also there are significant differences in the trienoic/tetrienoic ratio, during EFA deficiency, between different phospholipids: the ratio is much higher in PC and PI than in the other phospholipids. PC is actively exchanging with the plasma compartment, because it is located at the external face of the plasma membrane; whereas in PI, which has a very high turnover, presumably also fatty acids undergo a faster turnover. These dots indicate that there are different responses of different tissues and of different phospholipids in the same tissue to essential fatty acid deficiency. The different response of liver and other tissues to the administration of linoleic or to other unsaturated fatty acids in the diet is also seen when we compare the different response to an excess of linoleic acid in the diet.

In a study we carried out a few years ago [4], we fed either low or high linoleic acid to rabbits, and measured the polyunsaturated fatty acid observed in essential fatty acid deficiency may further influence the oxygenated pathways for the transformation of the polyunsaturates, since the oxygenages are active on the 20:3 n-9 generating different types of products.

In contrast to essential fatty acid deficiency situation, the administration of linoleic acid also affects in a different way the formation of eicosanoids. It has been shown that up to a certain percentage of the diet from 0 to 5 or 6% of the diet of the energy, linoleic acid enhances the formation of eicosanoids derived from arachidonic acid, on the other side it has been shown also, in our laboratory, that feeding rabbits [4] high levels of linoleic acid, around 10% of the energy (which is more or less the amount suggested by different organizations in order to counteract the effects of saturated fatty acids), the formation of eicosanoids is depressed. When very high levels of linoleic acid are fed in the diet, in fact, the content of arachidonic acid in tissues is actually reduced and this results in lower formation of arachidonic acid-derived eicosanoids.

The fatty acids derived from alphalinolenic, eicosapentanoic acid (20 carbons, with 5 double bonds), is also interfering very effectively with the arachidonic acid cascade. Both alphalinolenic and eicosapentanoic acid and all the fatty acids of the n-3 series can interfere with the metabolism of linoleic to arachidonic acid. In addition, there is also replacement of arachidonic acid by eicosapentanoic acid. Also the activity of the enzymes involved in the conversion of arachidonic acid to the eicosanoic products is affected by eicosapentanoic acid and, finally, products with biological activities different from those of the products derived from arachidonic acid are produced from this precursor.

Another aspect which may be important in considering the influences of essential fatty acids in the diet, on cell functions, is via modifications of the phospholipase activity which acts on the polyphosphoinositides and gives rise to two important second messengers. The activation of special receptors triggers the activation of a phospholipase C, through specific proteins. The diacylglycerol, which is produced after phospholipase C-activated break down of polyphosphoinositides, is involved in the activation of protein kinase C, whereas inositol phosphates, especially IP3, are responsible for the mobilisation of calcium in the cells. We have fed rabbits [6] for six weeks with diets rich in either oleic acid (olive oil), or rich in linoleic acid (corn oil) or rich in eicosapentaenoic acid (fish oil). We measured the consequence on platelets, not only aggregation and production of thromboxane or other eicosanoids but also the formation of the inositol phosphate products, which are also indicators of the activation of phospholipase C. At 10 seconds after stimulation, platelets from animals fed the three different diets produced different amounts of these products. Both the administration of fish oil and corn oil depressed the formation of IP3, which is the biologically active compound generated through this pathway.

In conclusion we can say that the administration of different amount and proportions of polyunsaturates of the linoleic and alphalinolenic acid series may modify different functional parameters through different parameters. Polyunsaturated fatty acids are in fact important constituents of the lipid phase of biological membrane. Each type of fatty acid has a specific role in modulating some of the functional parameters which we have previously discussed. The complexity of phospholipids in cell membranes is derived from basic metabolic requirements: maintenance of the barrier, maintenance of the physico-chemical environment that supports optimal membrane function, maintenance of phospholipid substrates that release arachidonic acid during cell stimulation and provision also of a reserve of polyunsaturates which is used by cells over short as well as long time periods.

Complex mechanisms operate to maintain the diversified and specialised distribution of polyunsaturates in cell lipid pools. But the availability of essential fatty acids in the diet affects the overall process. During development formation of new membranes is associated with growth processes in the tissue. Under these conditions maintenance of membrane properties and functions becomes a very critical homeostatic requirement. These combined requirements, for growth and maintenance, emphasize the necessity for an optimal supply both from a qualitative and quantitative point of view of the polyunsaturates of both the omega 6 and omega 3 series and these concepts of course apply directly to the formulation of optimal lipid supplements to the diet of neonates and infants.

I have finished and wish to thank you for your attention.

References

1. Sweet W.D., Scroeder F. (1988) *FEBS Letter* 229: 188-92.
2. Galli C., Agradi E., Paoletti R. (1975) *J Neurochem* 24: 1187-90.
3. Lefkowith J.B., Flippo V., Sprecher H., Needleman P. (1985) *J Biol Chem* 260: 5736-44.
4. Galli C., Agradi E., Petroni E. (1981) *Lipids* 16: 165-72.
5. Stubbs C.D., Smith A.D. (1984) *Biochim Biophys Acta* 779: 89-137.
6. Medini L., Colli S., Mosconi C., Colli S., Tremoli E. *Biochem Pharmacol* 39: 129-33.

Discussion

Chairman: Well, thank you, Prof Galli, for your interesting presentation. We have time for 5 minutes discussion, perhaps you have some questions to Prof Galli.

G. Béréziat: As you know, there are different pools in phospholipids in membranes and there is a different turnover rate. Could you say something about the possibility that there are also some different pools which can act as precursors for eicosanoids? When you have variations in the diet some pools may change and this change might not be the same in the production of eicosanoids.

C. Galli: Thank you for this question which is very important and I think it is very difficult to answer. There is some indirect evidence indicating that different pools of fatty acids may be utilized which can be differentially affected by the diet. One point which I want to make is that it has been shown that you may change the formation of eicosanoids in the body, after supplementation of different fatty acids, within very short periods of time, a few days, without even changing the composition of the membranes. So there is a suggestion that perhaps there is some specific fatty acid pool which is affected directly by the diet. This fatty acid pool might not be integrated into membrane structures, but they may act directly as precursors of the eicosanoids. Another indirect information which can be obtained through very simple *in vitro* studies is that if you, for instance, incubate different types of cells with a given mass of labelled arachidonic acid, they produce different proportions of labelled and unlabelled prostaglandins. When platelets are incubated with labelled arachidonate, for instance, both labelled and unlabelled thromboxane is formed. On the other side, when slices of brain tissue are incubated with labelled arachidonate, no labelled prostaglandin is produced, although cell phospholipids become highly labelled. At the same time, considerable amounts of unlabelled prostaglandins accumulate during the incubation. This indicates that in brain slices endogenous substrate released from tissue lipids is used for prostaglandin synthesis, and that there are two arachidonic acid pools: one is used for prostaglandin synthesis, and the other rapidly equilibrates with exogenous substrate. Platelets, instead, can convert directly the exogenous precursor to prostaglandins.
Now the question whether information from nutritional studies is adequate to establish which one of the components of the pools is affected more easily I think is very difficult to answer.

J. Ghisolfi: The biological effects of change in fatty acid composition are generally observed with very important differences in essential fatty intake. Have these changes been observed at different levels of linoleic acid intake, for instance, 1 to 6% of total calories as linoleic acid? Another question, you described the inhibition of delta 6 desaturase. What is the high level you have used in order to observe this desaturase inhibition?

C. Galli: We were not directly measuring desaturation reactions. I think it is difficult to extrapolate changes in the desaturation steps through the influence of dietary manipulations on the fatty acid composition of membranes. I think there are so many different processes of steps, desaturation is one aspect, but, also, the specific uptake of certain fatty acids and the transacylation reactions in cell membranes are more important than just the desaturation and elongation reactions. What we did was just feeding animals diets containing either 10% of the energy as linoleic acid or 2 to 3%. Then we observed in platelets and also in leucocytes a depletion of arachidonic acid and accumulation of precursors linoleic acid. But in the liver, this did not occur, indicating that desaturation is more important in the liver; but in other cells other types of processes are more important than desaturation.

Chairman: Just in connection with Prof Ghisolfi's question, may I have more information about these megadoses of linoleic acid? In your scale you show that there is negative effect on conversion of linoleic acid towards arachidonic acid and you said it is both a metabolic and a physiologic mechanism.

C. Galli: The question is about that term megadose, I don't know whether this can be applied properly. Many medical organizations suggest an optimal intake of about 7 to 10% of linoleic acid in the diet versus 10% saturated and 10% monounsaturated fatty acids. This is not far from the concentrations we have used. Now the question is that we were looking only to some specific aspects, formation of thromboxane, platelet aggregation and you cannot extrapolate from these data to the overall effects on various systems. What we can say is that if you feed high linoleic acid, in tissues where the eicosanoic cascade is very active, for instance, in platelets the cascade is depressed. This effect has been shown by other investigators too. We don't know whether this applies to other tissues which may have a different type of change in the balance of fatty acids in response to linoleic acid in the diet. I wish to stress that we did not really use a megadose, but rather a high dose of linoleic acid.

Chairman: That is a very important point and I think you will have the opportunity to speak again about this problem tomorrow during the round table. Thank you Prof Galli for this interesting presentation.

2

Essential fatty acids and brain development and function

J.M. BOURRE

INSERM U.26, Hôpital Fernand-Widal, 200, rue du Faubourg Saint-Denis, 75475 Paris Cedex 10, France

First I would like to thank very very much Prof Ghisolfi and Dr Putet for the energy they are spending in organising this meeting and also the different meetings on the polyunsaturated fatty acids. For various reasons I am also very glad this session is being chaired by Prof Crastes de Paulet.

Before presenting the results we have obtained mainly at the level of the alpha-linolenic acid, I would like to remind you of a few points which I feel to be very important in terms of brain structure and development. The first point is that brain development is genetically programmed, which means that when the once for all opportunity has gone it is extremely difficult to get any recovery. The second point is that cell renewal in the brain is extremely slow or even nil, for instance when some neurons or some oligodentrocytes have disappeared they are not replaced by another neuron or oligodendrocyte.

The following point is that renewal of the membranes (including neuronal membranes) is extremely slow. For example, in the myelin, the half life of some fatty acids is more than one year on the phospholipid; which means that when the phospholipid is in the membrane and when the fatty acids are in the phospholipids they are supposed to stay for a very long period of time. If non-physiological lipids are used in those phospholipids, these non-physiological fatty acids will make the membrane very fragile for a very long period of time. And the last point is that the brain tissue is the second tissue in terms of concentration of lipids, as it contains very high amounts of lipids, just after the adipose masses. In contrast with the adipose masses all these lipids are found in membranes, they are not used for energy to any extent.

On the first slide is presented an example of the very high activity during brain development. It shows you oligodendrocytes and the unfolded myelin, and this is in a very priveleged situation which is found in the optic nerve because sometimes, let's say for instance in the occipital lobe, one oligodendrocyte can myelinate as much as 50-100 axons. During the myelination and during the brain development these small cells, the oligodendrocytes, are able to synthesize many times, 5 times, their own weight in terms of membrane lipids; so one has to provide this cell the lipid it needs including polyunsaturated fatty acids. Because this membrane contains high amounts of saturated and monounsaturated fatty acids but also high amounts of polyunsaturated fatty acids in its lipids. So, if considering the fatty acids in the nervous tissue, you can see over here that in fact the polyunsaturated fatty acid does represent at minimum one third of the whole fatty acids in all the cells and organelles we have isolated (*Table I*). When considering the different polyunsaturated fatty acids it is interesting to note that in fact the precursors linoleic or alpha-linolenic acid are not present, all fatty acids which are present in the membranes in the nervous tissue are those very long chains from the n-6 series or from the n-3 series, mainly arachidonic acid and cervonic acid. The question was raised 5 or 6 years ago, what about the essentiality of alphalinolenic acid in terms of brain development and brain function? The first experiments we made were to feed an animal with the labelled alphalinolenic acid. After feeding the animal with this acid, the labelled activity is uptaken and found in cervonic acid, the label is heavily up-taken, this is obtained without any staining, this is just an autohistoradiography and you can see that cerebellum and also hippocampus and different brain regions are very easily determined with this technique.

Table I. Polyunsaturated fatty acids in nervous tissue

	% Total	% 20:4 (n-6)	% 22:6 (n-3)
Neurons	32	15	8
Nerve endings	33	18	12
Oligodendrocytes	20	9	5
Myelin	15	9	5
Astrocytes	29	10	11
Capillaries and microvessels	35	16	10
Mitochondria	30	18	10
Microsomes	29	11	10
Retina	45	5	35
Membrane (photoreceptors)	65	4	56
Peripheral nerve	10	7	2
Schwann cells	22	11	5

What about the effect of feeding animal different diets?

In fact we have fed animals two kinds of diet. One group of rats was fed either rapeseed oil or soybean oil, and another group of rats was fed sunflower oil or eventually nut oil. Sunflower oil was compared to soybean oil and nut oil was compared to rapeseed oil. When in the diet the amount of alpha-linolenic was reduced by let's say 25-34, then the end product in the membrane was reduced at maximum by two times (*Table II*), so in fact the cell which was the most protected in the whole organism was the neuron because a 25 times reduction in the diet provoked a twofold reduction in the neurons. All the other organelles of cells or organs we looked for presented a defect in cervonic acid, which was totally compensated by 22:5 n-6, a fatty acid which was first described by Claudio Galli and this fatty acid having 22 carbon atoms, 5 double bond but from the n-6 series. So one molecule of cervonic acid was replaced by one of these molecules.

Table II. Levels of 22:6 (n-3) and 22:5 (n-6) in rats fed a diet deficient in alpha-linolenic acid

	22:6 (n-3)	22:5 (n-6)
Neurons	48	214
Nerve endings	27	1 088
Oligodendrocytes	10	240
Myelin	14	1 200
Astrocytes	47	344
Capillaries	26	362
Mitochondria	25	917
Microsomes	28	592
Retina	36	1 280
Sciatic nerve	28	1 000
$\dfrac{(n-3)^-}{(n-3)^+} \times 100$		

What about the speed of the recovery, *figure 1* shows what happens if feeding the animal a deficient diet and now, when being 60 days of age, feeding the animal with a non-deficient diet. In other words these animals were previously fed a sunflower oil diet and then when being 60 days old they were changed to a soybean oil diet. You can see that for the neurons, for the athrocytes, for the oligodendrocytes, within a two to three months period the recovery is not totally obtained, which means that the speed of the recovery is extremely slow in the brain, in contrast with the liver. In the liver within two or three weeks the composition in terms of cervonic acid is totally normal; rather surprising was to find out that the brain capillaries and minor vessels from the brain also presented a very slow recovery, which was unexpected because in fact these cells are in the presence of normal lipoproteins which are synthesized by the liver which is returned to a normal composition. So, these cells behave like the rest of the brain and not like the rest of the organisms, which raise many questions in terms of recovery and in terms of transport of polyunsaturated fatty acids through the blood brain barrier.

What about the effect of this efficiency in cervonic acid which is compensated by 22:5 and 22:6 series on membrane structure and function? The fluidity of the

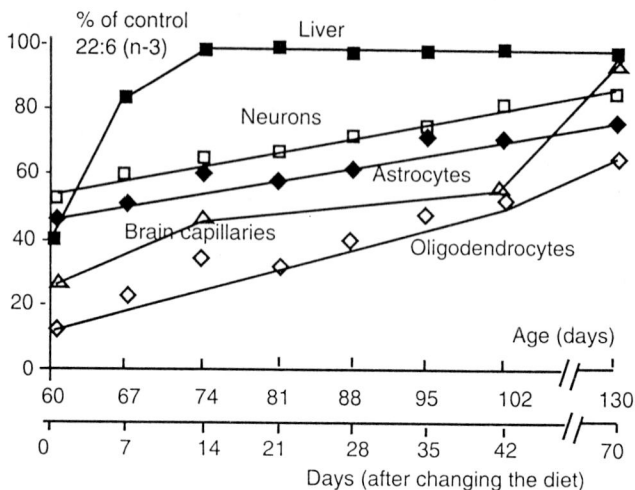

Figure 1. Speed of recovery.

membrane is heavily affected, and, interestingly, the fluidity of the membrane is affected at the level of the non-polar region, but also at the level of the polar region. This was obtained in nerve endings, and we found the same, for instance, in the red blood cells (*Table III*).

Table III. Alteration of membrane fluidity nerve endings

	$(n-3)^+$	$(n-3)^-$	
DPH (Apolar region)	0.333±0.004	0.320±0.001	−4%
TMA-DPH (polar region)	0.352±0.001	0.359±0.002	+2%
PROP-DPH (polar region)	0.360±0.001	0.370±0.003	+3%

Besides the fluidity some enzymatic activities are also affected (*Table IV*). It was previously shown by Prof Galli that ATPase was affected in the liver; it is also heavily affected in the nerve endings. One has to remember that the brain represents 2% of the body weight in the adult but in fact it uses 20% of the energy and half of this energy is used by only this enzyme, so it means that 10% of the energy which is used by the whole organism is used only by one enzyme in the brain which is APTase. This enzymatic activity is reduced nearly by 40% in the nerve endings. Another enzyme is 5′ nucleotidase and this enzyme which is found in membrane is also reduced but slightly less reduced, it is reduced by 40% in the whole brain and this is in agreement with studies by Bersons showing that in fact this enzyme 5′

nucleotidase is controlled only by the alpha-linolenic series but not by the linoleic series. What he did was to feed animals a controlled diet and then the activity was 100%, feeding animals a fat deficient diet then the activity was dramatically reduced and if feeding these animals with linoleic acid then there was no recovery in the enzymatic activity. In contrast, if feeding the animals with alpha-linolenic acid the total recovery was obtained, which means that this enzyme and the enzymatic activity is controlled only by alpha-linolenic acid. Besides alteration at the level of the composition of the fluidity enzymatic activity we found that in fact also some function could be affected such as the electroretinogram. If comparing sunflower fed animal and soybean fed animal, then to get the same electrophysiological signal one has to give the deficient animal a light which is tenfold more potent, which means they present a huge deficiency in terms of vision. Very curiously this deficiency disappears during development and ageing, although the biochemical abnormality is still present.

Table IV. Activities of brain enzymes in rats fed an alpha-linolenic deficient diet

	Brain	Myelin	Nerve endings
5′-nucleotidase	0.70	0.74	1.2
Na^+K^+ATPase	0.95	1.10	0.55
CNPase	0.95	0.78	0.00
Values are ratio of enzyme activities in $(n-3)^-$ compared to $(n-3)^+$ diets			

Besides the electroretinogram, some learning performances are heavily affected, this being seen with a shuttle box test which is to put an animal in a big cage. This cage is divided into two parts, there is a hole between the two parts. In one part we put the animal, we turn on the light and 15 seconds afterwards we send electricity in the cage and the animal has to escape to the other part of the cage. The number of non-passages meaning that the animal is just looking for the light and then receives electricity, doing strictly nothing, is like somewhat idiotic. The number of non-passages is much more important in sunflower fed animals in comparison with soybean fed animals. This is not due to the fact that these animals have impaired vision because some other tests such as the open field are totally normal or nearly normal, so it means that this effect is really due to deficiency in learning. The question which is raised is, are these animals more fragile? This is one test we have done which was to measure the susceptibility of the animal to a neurotoxine such as TTT, triethyltin: the sunflower fed animals die much more rapidly (*figure 2*). This is a combined mortality after injecting this toxine to the animal. Considering another toxine which is much more popular, at least in France, and even in this country, which is alcohol, the fluidising effect on the membrane is different on nerve endings (we found also the same on the red blood cells). It is not the same if feeding the animal with soybean oil or sunflower oil.

Finally, if considering the blood brain barrier, this barrier is extremely solid and extremely efficient. Very curiously, if feeding an animal a diet which was deficient in alpha-linolenic acid then we found that in some brain regions we had some leaks

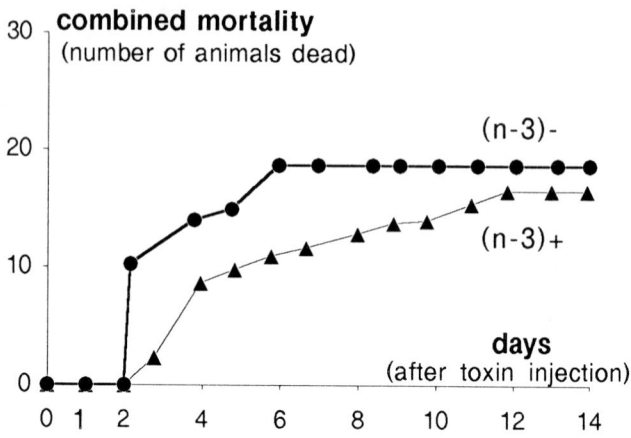

Figure 2. Acute toxicity (triethyltin) 7 µl/kg.

which were shown diffusing for instance saccharose, saccharose is normally nearly not uptaken by the brain or poorly uptaken by the brain, and if feeding the animal a diet deficient in alpha-linolenic acid the saccharose uptake was much more uptaken in some regions but not in others. It means that a diet deficient in alpha-linolenic acid provokes some leaks in the blood brain barrier which is very interesting in terms of transport of drugs for instance, which could be dramatic in terms of transport of toxines. We are currently doing some studies in this field.

The next question was what about the quantity which has to be given to the animal in terms of alpha-linolenic acids so as to get a normal or a so-called normal brain development and a normal brain function. What we have done was to feed animals increasing amounts of alpha-linolenic acid by mixing nut oil and rapeseed oil, or by mixing sunflower oil and soybean oil. We found (*figure 3*) that if increasing the amount of alpha-linolenic acid in a diet then we increased the amount of cervonic acid in the brain, in the nerve endings, the retina, the myelin and the sciatic nerve up to a certain amount which was something around 0.4% of the calories. Over this quantity it was a plateau which means that increasing the amount of alpha-linolenic acid in a diet did not provoke any accumulation of these fatty acids or its longer chains in brain structures. Looking at the other organs it was really interesting to note that in fact the same thing was obtained in the brain, this is the same curve, in the liver, in the heart then at this level which is at around 0.4% of the calorie, instead of having a plateau then we found just a change in the slope of the curve. So, we could propose that in fact the minimum amount of alphalinolenic acid to be found in the diet is 0.4% of the calories. But the question is what about the minimum amount to be found in the diet for linoleic acid, as it is known that in fact the utilization of alpha-linolenic acid could be changed if increasing the amount of linoleic acid in the diet. In fact if changing the amount of linoleic acid in the diet,

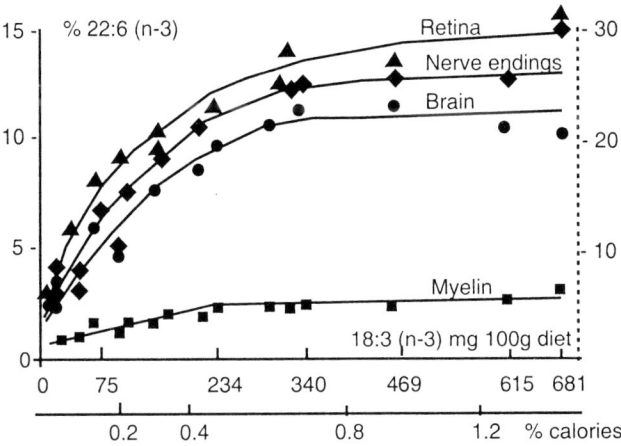

Figure 3. Relationship between dietary alpha-linolenic acid and cervonic acid level in nervous tissue.

but not giving megadose to the animal, it does not change dramatically the amount of alpha-linolenic acid series in the membrane. If feeding animals increasing amounts of linoleic acid in the diet, very curiously the minimum amounts of linoleic acid which are needed by the brain are small, because as low as 0.3% of the calories of linoleic acid was sufficient to obtain a plateau in arachidonic acid, which means that in fact this arachidonic acid in the brain is heavily controlled. As soon as a minimum quantity is found in the diet the brain actively uptakes this linoleic acid so as to maintain this very important fatty acid in the phospholipid. In contrast in the other organs then the plateau was obtained at a different level. For the liver it was obtained for 2.4% of the calories, nearly the same value was found for the lung, for the kidney, much less was necessary for the testis and for the muscle. So, in fact the minimum amount to be found in the diet in terms of alpha-linolenic acid is 0.4% of the calories and the minimum amount for linoleic acid is 2.4% of the calories. This is in rat and this is in developing rat. The question is which kind of oil to add in the salad cream mixed meal. The only oils containing doses of the two essential fatty acids are the rapeseed oil and soybean oil, for ecologists I would add walnut oil or wheat germ oil.

But in fact there is another important question which is what about the usefulness of fish oil. This oil is very important in terms of preventive treatment of cardio-vascular disease. It is also nutriously interesting because all membranes, including the brain membranes, the fatty acids which are present are not the precursors of linoleic and alpha-linolenic acid but the longer chains which are arachidonic acid and cervonic acid. One used to say that desaturase affected during certain diseases even during ageing which has not been proved until now, and it could be interesting to feed mammals directly with the long chains and not with the precursors. In fact, one has to consider that it could be interesting because what we did was to raise, to grow the cells *in vitro,* to make some cell culture and on this cell culture we were able to get cells which these brain cells were able to differentiate, to divide and to release and to uptake neuron mediators only if the cells were grown in the presence of the long chains and not at all in the presence of the shorter chains, either one of them or two of them. So at least *in vitro* using cell culture the fatty acids which are essential for the brain could be the long chains not the precursors, so the question is raised from where those precursors are coming.

Are they synthesized very actively and very rapidly in the brain, are they synthesized or are they uptaken, selectively uptaken, at the level of the blood brain barrier? Are they synthesized in the liver or are they coming from the diet? This is an unsolved question for the moment. But anyway for the brain it seems the essential fatty acids could be the long chains, so it could be interesting to feed the animal fish oils. In fact, one has to consider those fish oils are interesting at three levels which are first nutrition, but also pharmacology, and then toxicology. And although being "a natural product", those fatty acids from the fish oils, if fed to the animals in excess could provoke some toxological effects. Some preliminary studies we have done show that if feeding the animals cod liver oil or salmon oil even added with tocopherol (ten times or fifteen times the dose which is proposed in humans), the level of arachidonic acid is reduced and conversely the level of cervonic acid is increased. It must be taken into account that slight changes at the level of the fatty acid composition of the membrane could change the fatty acid composition of the brain membrane, the electrophysiology and the overall function of the organ.

So one has to be very careful with those fish oils because if changing the fatty acid composition in the brain then I would expect that some subtle changes in the brain function can occur. So, in fact these fish oils are very interesting for two reasons, the first reason being that EPA is interesting for controlling cardio-vascular diseases and also because those fish oils provide cervonic acid. But I would say, for artificial food and for the formulas, it's probably not a good idea to give the baby in the same time EPA and cervonic acid because EPA is reducing the level of the synthesis of triglycerides.

So, to get neurons having a good function we have to provide those neurons and we have to provide all the brain cells. I remind you of the fact that the brain is let's say 1.4 kg and just between 10-15 % of the brain weight is devoted to the neurons, 150 g for the neurons and the rest is something else. So we have to take care with the rest of the brain which is the non-neuronal part of the brain and to get a good neuronal development, a good neuronal function, one has to feed the mammal with the polyunsaturated fatty acid from the two series which are the n-6 series and the n-3 series.

But at the same time I must remind that it is very important to protect those fatty acids against peroxidation, especially in the brain because this organ uses huge amounts of oxygen and the renewal of the cell is nil and the renewal of membrane is extremely slow although containing huge amounts of polyunsaturated fatty acid. So, one has to be careful with those polyunsaturated fatty acids, they need a protection against peroxidation, which is provided by tocopherol. It is renewed by some other system which is largely unknown for the moment and those systems containing vitamin C but also glutathione peroxidases with selenium and various super-oxides.

All these studies have been made in animal because in fact it's totally impossible to get any result in humans for evident ethical reasons. It's not possible to feed the human with different diets, and then to perform some biopsies from the brain or even from the liver, to decide if those different diets have changed the brain composition, the membrane composition and the membrane function. Thank you very much for your attention.

Discussion

Chairman: I think that everybody is convinced that you gave a very beautiful lecture, I thank you again and I use my privilege of President to keep the discussion open during 10 minutes because it is very interesting to have a discussion after your presentation, it was very important, very humouristic too, you bring many results but you also bring many questions. The discussion is open.

B. Koletzko: Thank you for your very stimulating presentation as is to be expected of you. I have three questions. You showed an interesting slide on the effect of alpha-linolenic acid supplementation on the learning behaviour in young rats. Your subsequent work did not really confirm their first results and would you comment on this controversy.
The second question. I noticed in your slides and abstract that you expressed your results as milligram fatty acid for a hundred grams of food, I assume that you probably took care to keep the level of fat intake and energy intake constant, but is there any reason why you would prefer the sixth version or the traditional expression of fatty acid intake as the percentage of energy intake? And the third question is, did you have any indication that intake of polyunsaturates influenced monounsaturated fatty acid content in the brain of your animals which is of course very high?

J.M. Bourre: OK so we have three questions and we've got 10 minutes. I will take the reverse, the last point, this is a very interesting point regarding the control of the polyunsaturated fatty acid composition in membrane including in the brain if changing the amount of oleic acid in the diet, that's right? In fact we have not done such experiments, the only thing we have done was feeding animals either nut oil or sunflower oil or linseed oil or soybean oil which contain different amounts of oleic acid, and we have never seen any difference between all those four diets, which means that the brain from all four groups of animals presented the same amount of monounsaturated fatty acids.
The following point was, what about expressing the results in per cent of calories, instead of milligram per 100 grams of food, so I do not know because I am more of a neuro-chemist and I have to adapt to the different ways of expressing the result according to your suggestion. I try now to speak in per cent of calories, which is easier to be presented, at least in English in a conference, and, also, I think it is more important for people to know in per cent of calories, because I feel it is more interesting to express results this way.
And the last question was the controversy about learning performances in these animals. So, I do not have any response for this kind of question except that in fact

if looking at the brain one has to be extremely careful because the brain is extremely resistant to any changes. So it means if you change the diet within a short period of time in the adults but not in the developing animal then you will not see any change or very poor changes in the brain. So it means all these studies were conducted with two groups of rats fed through generations either one type of diet or another type of diet, because if you feed an animal sunflower oil, if changing the diet within two or three months it will be very difficult to have stabilised changes in all parts of the brain, so within two weeks or within three weeks you will be able to see slight changes in some part of the brain, but within two months some other regions will not have changed. So those differences might be due to the fact that there were some differences at the level of the diet. If feeding the animal for a short period of time you will probably see some changes at the level of the fatty acid but you will not be able to see some changes at the level of enzymatic activities or in the learning performances. So I would say that in fact studies are now conducted in Toronto, by Caroll on the learning performances of the animal fed different diets, and she found very interesting results on the learning performances of the animals. Moreover, animals fed diets deficient in alpha-linolenic acid were less susceptible to pain. So, I remind you that we choose the shuttle box test to avoid visual problems in the animal and to be sure it was learning performances which were affected and the control was the open field. But in fact it could be possible that these animals are less susceptible to pain which means if they do not escape to the other part of the cage, it could be due to the fact that they are less susceptible to the pain, so the discussion is open to these "learning performances". But I would say that in fact it is totally sure that there are some problems at the level of learning performances, whatever the model, and it has been shown recently by Okurama's group in Japan, with the same type of experiments.

The test was to push a button 15 seconds after the light switched on to obtain food, so the deficient animal had presented a longer period of time to understand that after the light was switched on they had to press the button to get the food.

Within two or three or four series of tests they finished by understanding the rule of the game, and if the technicians changed the rule of the game (when the light was switched on it was not possible to obtain the food), then the control animals were very rapidly able to understand that the rule of the game had been changed but in contrast the deficient animals were not able to understand.

So, it takes a longer time to understand and it also takes a longer time to extinguish what they have learnt previously.

Chairman: I think it's time for the last question, Dr Galli.

C. Galli: You have shown a relationship between the amount of alpha-linolenic acid in the diet and the accumulation of cervonic acid. Now the question is you have been using different mixtures of oils, do you feel the absolute amounts of linoleic/linolenic acid are essential or also the proportional ratio of these fatty acids in the diet, that they interfere with the activation of the given amount of alphalinolenic?

J.M. Bourre: So it means that we have something else to do. In fact both things are very important. The level of cervonic acid is not heavily affected when increasing the amount of linoleic acid in the diet. In fact if feeding animals different amounts of linoleic acid, from 2.2% to 10% of the calories. So, if standing the diet in terms of linoleic acid, in the same way the minimum amount of alpha-linolenic acid which was needed was between 0.25% of the calories up to 0.30% of the calories, which means if you multiply by 5 the amount of linoleic acid the amount of alpha-linolenic acid which is needed is increased by, let's say, 10%, so it's not very, very important. So, in fact the minimum amount and the actual quantity is important. If feeding the animal high amounts of oil, sunflower oil, the linoleic acid/alpha-linolenic acid ratio is dramatically high. Then you have two processes in the same time which is too high amount of linoleic acid, so you increase the amount of 22:5 n-6 and reduce the amount of alpha-linolenic acid, which provokes the same thing which is increasing 22:5 n-6. Both things are important in fact.

Chairman: Your last question.

J. Rey: You have shown that you obtain a plateau with increasing the level of n-3 or n-6 series in the brain and different organs; what are your reasons for thinking that this plateau is an optimal value?

J.M. Bourre: I had the same question two weeks ago, I have no response. Defining normality is always difficult, we have to start with something. As far as a plateau is obtained, then it's supposed to be the optimum value; also it could be considered as being the optimum value because the same level of fatty acid is obtained whatever the diet: if feeding the animal vegetable oils or fish oils, the plateau is obtained at the same level.

Chairman: Dr Putet, I think that is the last question.

G. Putet: You said that over 0.4% of the linolenic acid intake as kilocalories, it is observed abnormalities in erythrocyte fatty acid distribution. Did you have the same type of abnormalities in omega 3 derivatives in the brain?

J.M. Bourre: Yes, one has to consider that we are not rats, but in fact if you take a corresponding piece of brain in the rat and of brain in the human, I mean not the frontal lobe, but some other region, the fatty acid composition is exactly the same. The brain weight in the human is higher and human is doing more brain during a longer period of time. Thus if those values are actually the good ones for the developing rat, they must be at least the values which have to be proposed for the human. So if being 0.4% of the calories for the rat it must be at least 0.4% of the calories for the human.

G. Putet: You said that rats when they were getting more aged recovered their visual function, but that the histological lesions of the retina were still present. How can you explain this fact?

J.M. Bourre: I don't have any comments for that and this is a very important point because in fact, as you know, the retina and specially the phospholipids in the retina contain huge amounts of cervonic acid (up to 80% in phosphatidylethanolamine). So in the retina this cervonic acid is replaced by 22.5 and n-6 and this biochemical abnormality is maintained all through the life of the animal. If you continue to feed the animal with a deficient diet of course, very curiously, although biochemical abnormality is continuously found, then the electro-physiological abnormality is corrected.

Chairman: Well, thank you, I think that we must stop now in spite of very interesting questions we have to ask you but we have time during the coffee break. Thank you again.

3

Essential fatty acid composition of tissue lipids in the perinatal period

M.T. CLANDININ, J. VAN AERDE

University of Alberta, Faculty of Medicine, Nutrition and Metabolism Research Group, 533 Newton Research Building, Edmonton, Alberta, Canada

First let me thank the organizers for providing me with this wonderful opportunity to come to Greece. If we can have the first slide I would like to provide a different perspective on essential fatty acid metabolism and provide you with the basis for the whole body estimations that we've made of infant essential fatty acid requirements for nutrients and some of the assumptions that have been made about how you determine what nutrients to feed. The traditional approach has considered the fats provided by milk through the cellular biology of the mammary gland as representative of the nutrients which meet the needs of the newborn infant. This certainly has been the case for many nutrients and is applicable to the normal term infant. This assumption is weak in terms of logic if you apply it to the premature infant, but we can derive specific information by analysis of the composition of milk, and by then relating this information to the fat composition of infant growth we can begin to make some generalizations. To assess the composition of infant growth, the accretion of fat in the infant both in the intra-uterine period and the extra-uterine period has to be considered. Growth of the premature infant presents special problems. For example, do we achieve extra-uterine growth of the premature infant in a manner that mimics the intra-uterine body composition in terms of some of the critical tissues such as brain?

To define the requirements of the newborn infant for fat we have to consider milk composition, tissue fat composition, fat absorption and fat oxidation to make some assumptions.

Milk content of long chain polyenoic EFAs

By the time lactation has matured about day 16 to 37 human milk contains around 1.5% of the fat as omega-6 fatty acids of C20 and C22 chain length. By the time lactation matures the level in pre-term versus term milk is essentially similar, and is approximately 1.5% of the total fatty acids. For C20 and C22 omega-3 the number is approximately 0.5 to 0.6% of the fatty acids so that milk contains a significant level of C20 and C22 omega-6 and omega-3 acids. Human milk also contains a whole range of other fatty acids. We have used analysis of milk from milks at day sixteen lactation from mothers delivering premature infants to estimate the infants essential fatty acid intake. By basing the level of milk intake at 200 ml per kg body weight of the infant, the amount of different fatty acids that the infant would receive can be calculated to provide a quantitative estimate of how much fatty acid a 1.3 kg premature infant would receive. Approximately a third of the fatty acid is saturated, another third is monoenes, about 850 mg of fatty acid per day being omega-6 and 140 mg/day being omega-3 fatty acids. The intake provides approximately 36 mg per day as arachidonic acid with at least an equivalent amount of other chain elongated-desaturated omega-6 fatty acids, and about 24 mg per day of docosahexaenoic acid.

Accretion of fats in different organs in the body

The estimated intra-uterine tissue accretion of omega-6 and omega-3 acids is dominated by accretion of these essential fatty acids in the adipose organ. This last trimester in the human is the time in which the adipose organ is built, and so there is tremendous growth in the adipose organ. The adipose tissue during this period has a high water content and is fairly cellular material containing a significant amount of essential fatty acid. During the early weeks of life the content of linoleic acid goes up as the linoleic acid intake in infants is increased through oral intake. We've also represented this through use of data that were published by investigators prior to 1984. The adipose tissue 18:2 content can be expressed as a function of dietary 18:2 intake. Liver presents a different situation. As body weight increases liver weight in grams per kg of body weight decreases, thus the liver represents a declining proportion of the total body weight as a potential reserve of essential fatty acid that could be drawn on. In the last trimester the liver's content of omega-6 C20 and C22 acids on a body weight basis is highest early during this period and declines as the liver per body weight decreases. The liver has a significant amount of these fatty acids during the early period of development and as the body grows, representing a declining ability to provide these from any amount that would be stored in some form. Arachidonic acid is stored and is higher in the liver during the last trimester. During the extra-uterine period this fatty acid seems to be moved out of the liver.

If we consider the accretion rates of the long chain polyenoics during the last trimester of development, we have 30 mg of omega-6 per week in brain, about 14 to 15 mg per week of omega-3, and with the largest amount of omega-3 and 6 going into the adipose tissue. The pattern of change in brain content of long chain polyenoic fatty acids is important. During the last trimester of gestation the levels of linoleic acid and linolenic acid in brain tend to be quite low. The main omega-6 and omega-3 constituents to occur are the chain elongated and desaturated forms. During the last trimester of development there is significant accretion of arachidonic and docosahexaenoic acids which are not continued until sometime after birth. We have been responsible for questioning whether the accretion of the chain-elongated polyunsaturated components in the brain of the premature infant could be derived from endogenous synthesis.

The basis question is then whether or not premature infants require nutritional support with very long chain polyunsaturated essential fatty acids. If infants are fed the chain elongated-desaturated component, the infant will incorporate these fatty acids into the plasma phospholipids, cholesterol esters and red blood cell membrane lipids. When the chain-elongated fatty acid is not fed, the levels of both arachidonic and particularly docosahexaenoic acids fall. We don't know the degree to which these changes that occur in the plasma lipid reflect what happens in tissues such as brain. Thus we don't have some of the essential answers to deduce whether feeding with long chain polyunsaturated fatty acid-supplemented formulas is required or not. The assumption that the composition of plasma red cell may mimic the composition of changes occurring in the brain still needs to be addressed. It is however reasonable to assume that plasma phospholipid polyunsaturated fatty acid content may reflect what the liver is producing.

We have been working on the development and regulation of enterocyte desaturase activities. In the animal model there is a significant amount of chain elongation-desaturation of essential fatty acid going on in the brush border in the enterocyte. Based on our results we know that the activity in the enterocyte relative to liver is approximately half if you express it on a per mg basis of what is found in the liver. Actually when the amount of intestinal mucosa is considered it is apparent that the intestinal mucosa is a relatively big organ in terms of modifying essential fatty acids absorbed and exporting them as chain elongated-desaturated products through the lipoprotein compartments to other parts of the body.

The entry of fatty acid to brain, the degree to which and forms in which the brain can take up polyunsaturated chain-elongated fatty acid is also an area that needs to be addressed.

Absorption of fat

We have examined the absorption of different fatty acids by premature infants fed human milk or formula. We have found that absorption of saturated fats is not as high as the absorption of polyunsaturated fats. Depending on how the infant is supplemented with calcium the absorption of fat is also reduced by formation of calcium soaps. A fundamentally different pattern of absorption exists for different fatty acids in the diet. Polyunsaturated fats seem to be absorbed with a coefficient of absorption of a least 90% and when stool fats from infants fed milk are examined no very long chain-desaturated products can be found. In these very young infants that are 4 or 5 days old, the bacterial flora is not very active and the polyunsaturated fats are not excreted, thus the basic assumption that these polyunsaturated fatty acids are very well absorbed is reasonable. Let us assume that the coefficient of absorption for essential fatty acids is at least 90% to make some basic calculations to estimate the fat and essential fatty acid intake required for growth of the premature infant. The maintenance energy would be about 80 kcal per kg for premature infants per day, the energy intake would be 120 kcal per kg, and the assumption that about half the available calories in milk is fat and that the coefficient of fat absorption is about 90%. This applies to the polyunsaturated fats and of course it doesn't apply for all the fats in the diet of the premature infant. Then with these assumptions, about 3.4 g of fat per day would be utilized for growth in the preterm infant in terms of tissue synthesis. There are other ways of calculating this number where you can come up with a number that is higher depending on the feeding situation. With those basic assumptions and numbers and with the caveat that the essential fatty acid is not preferentially conserved from beta oxidation (this is a weakness which would reduce the numbers projected for we do know from studies in adults that certain fatty acids are more preferred substrates for fat oxidation than are others) by group. With that basic idea the preterm infant's essential fatty acid requirement would be something around the order of 1 100 mg of omega-6 fatty acids per day and 140 mg of omega-3 per day assuming that approximately 17 g of body weight gain per day occurs. The appropriate balance may be the best way to look at the dietary intake rather than as the absolute amount. It is our estimate that linoleic acid intake should be about 12% of fatty acids with about 1% being the 18:3 omega-3. In terms of the C20 and C22 omega-6, what amounts would provide the physiological intake that is comparable to the intake from human milk? In this regard, about 1% for the C20 and C22 omega-6, and about 0.6 or 0.7% for the omega-3 fatty acids would be appropriate. The balance between the C20 and C22 omega-6 to omega-3 fatty acids is most important and should approximate about 1.4 to 1.5.

Discussion

Chairman: Thank you very much Dr Clandinin for the very important data concerning the question and the need for polyunsaturated fatty acids in the foetus and preterm infant, but I think that we have a lot of questions.

G. Putet: I want to ask you some questions about the composition of the term infant during the first 12 weeks of age when you studied them and studied the brain composition. As feeding is very important what was the feeding of these infants? Were they fed formulas or human milk?

M.T. Clandinin: Well, your point is a good one and it's actually why we have stayed away from that area of the problem. We have emphasized in everything we have done the intra-uterine period in the first weeks of life simply because we are unable to really make any reasonable assessment about intakes. The protocol we had for the infants we studied for tissue composition was such that we were fairly certain the infants were growing normally up until the time of death, so the only assumption you could make is that the infants were growing normally. The causes of death for the infants at that later period were automobile accidents for several of them, but actually most of them were sudden infant death, so even these were apparently normal up until the time of death. Past that it's not possible to make any sort of valid conclusions of what their intakes were. Thus we have tended to stay away from any kind of analysis or assumptions that were based upon composition of infants living after the immediate post partum period.

G. Putet: I understand that about the amount, but do you know if they were breast fed or formula fed?

M.T. Clandinin: We do and think they were a heterogeneous group in this regard. I would have to check as it was ten years ago that we collected the information.

J. Rey: I will briefly return to normal growth. Those babies who died at 12 weeks, you can obtain a normal growth with any kind of diet even with absolutely no amount of essential fatty acids, so you need to have more information on the diet of these babies. It's very difficult for me to follow your calculation of requirements and perhaps we shall discuss this later, but my question is, what is the influence of the mother's diet on fatty acid accretion during pregnancy, have you any idea of this?

M.T. Clandinin: Well even though I think it's a good question, I don't think that we have good information on it. There's probably some animal model information on the effect of diet on composition of foetal tissues. I'm not intimately familiar with it and I don't think a great deal done, so I don't think the ultimate answer to your question exists.

B. Salle: I had exactly the same question as Dr Rey. My second question is about the absorption of fatty acid. Are you sure of the difference in absorption of $C16$,

C18, etc., Dr Clandinin: the difference between human milk and formula, that's right. How do you feed your preterm babies? Do you use their own mother's milk, pasteurized milk or raw milk?

M.T. Clandinin: Yes, we've published this data in quite a bit of detail. Basically my answer to your question is the infants are fed their own mother's milk and it's not pasteurized.

D. Hull: I'm pursuing the same question about maternal diet and foetal growth. On the data that you gave us do you have any idea on what the mothers were on average eating? I mean F. Wildousan from her studies suggested that if mothers were eating a high amount of essential fatty acids there was more in the foetus at term than if mothers were fed lower amounts of essential fatty acids. Do you have any information?

M.T. Clandinin: No, unfortunately the kind of information you allude to simply could not have been obtained.

D. Hull: Where in fact does the habit come to increase in diet amount of essential fatty acids, had that already taken over Canada when you did your study or not?

M.T. Clandinin: I think that the only assumption that you could make is not a very strong or a particularly reliable one. Our fat intakes in Canada tend to be high with a P/S intake of approximately 0.4.

Chairman: Dr Clandinin, may I ask you a question? You mentioned the problem of betaoxidation. It is an important question because you have no data at all at that time and if you occult this problem it is very difficult to give a conclusion on the metabolism and the fate of any fatty acid. Have you some idea how to proceed to go further in this vital question?

M.T. Clandinin: We're doing this on an on-going basis in adults. We have now started studies in neonates to assess the problem. Dr John VanAerde has set up a piglet model which is primarily intravenous to determine how different conditions alter the whole body oxidation of essential fatty acid.

Chairman: Have you used stable isotopes to label the fatty acids?

M.T. Clandinin: We're doing stable isotope experiments now on adults. We have also chosen to work out the neonatal problem, first using the piglet and then applying the design to the premature infant. As you know, there are many complexities involved and that's why we've gone through the piglet first.

SESSION II

Chairman: Susan CARLSON (USA)

4

Effects of current infant formula on brain and retinal lipid development. Effect of formula with 2% 18:3 n–3 on n–6 and n–3 fatty acid status of low birthweight infants

Sheila M. INNIS

University of British Columbia, B.C. Children's Hospital, Research Center, Shaughnessy Site, 950 - West 28th Avenue, Vancouver, British Columbia, Canada V5Z4HA, Canada

First let me add my thanks to the organizers and Milupa, along with those of the previous speakers this morning, for inviting me to this beautiful city and to participate in these meetings.

I would like to focus my attention in this paper on the results of studies which are part of a research programme we are undertaking on the essential fatty acid requirements of the newborn, particularly with regard to a possible requirement for carbon chain 20 and 22 fatty acids. Several publications have appeared in the literature to demonstrate that infants fed formula have higher levels of linoleic acid 18:2 n–6, and lower levels of the carbon chain 20 and 22 n–6 and n–3 fatty acids in their plasma and red blood cell phospholipids than breast fed infants. Several possible reasons may explain these differences between infants fed formula and those fed breast milk. These include an inability of the newborn to desaturate 18:2 n–6 and 18:3 n–3, inhibition of desaturation for example by inappropriate fatty acid balance, or an inadequate level of 18:3 n–3 in the formula. Another possibility which I will not discuss at this workshop is the effects of differences in lipoprotein and cholesterol metabolism between the formula and breast fed infant.

The essential question of course is whether the n–6 and/or n–3 carbon chain 20 and 22 fatty acids in breast milk are essential nutrients for the infant. This question asks if the infant is unable to desaturate dietary 18:2 n–6 and/or 18:3 n–3 at a sufficient rate to supply the long chain polyenoics. By the term long chain polyenoics

I mean the carbon chain 20 and 22 n–6 and n–3 fatty acids (abbreviated as LCP in the *figures*) needed for structural lipid accretion. The approach we have taken has been to determine whether or not there may be a limitation of desaturation, rather than immaturity of desaturase activities, in neonates fed formula. The regulation of the desaturase enzymes has been addressed already by Dr Galli and Dr Bourre. Briefly, the activity of the desaturase enzymes with a specific n–6 or n–3 fatty acid substrate is related both to the level of the substrate fatty acids, and to the supply of the product and competing fatty acids. For example, delta-6-desaturase activity appears to be increased at low levels of 18:2 n–6 but suppressed by high concentrations of 18:2 n–6, as well as by the desaturation products of both the n–6 and n–3 series fatty acids. The questions which we have addressed can be summarized as:

1. Do infants require a preformed dietary source of carbon chain 20 and 22 n–6 and/or n–3 fatty acids because desaturase enzyme activity is low in the perinatal period?

2. What is the effect of current formula lipids which do not contain carbon 20 and 22 n–6 and/or n–3 fatty acids on brain structural lipid accretion and associated brain membrane functions in the neonate?

I'm going to start with the second question first. This we have attempted to answer in piglets fed formulas of different fat composition. In these studies we have looked at whether or not the changes in the brain fatty acids of piglets fed formula similar to infant formula indicate immature desaturation. In this case, the levels of both the long chain polyenoic n–6 and n–3 fatty acids would be expected to decrease. Alternatively, an increase in one series and decrease in the other series of long chain polyenoic fatty acids would be interpreted as evidence of an inbalanced or deficient fat blend. We have also addressed the important question of whether or not plasma and red blood cell phospholipid fatty acids adequately reflect the diet-induced changes occurring in the brain and retinal lipid. There are several reasons why piglets were selected for study; these include the close similarity in the timing of the brain growth spurt in the pig relative to man. The maximum period of brain growth when related to perinatal age is about similar in humans and pigs, extending from the beginning of the last trimester of gestation, to peak about the time of normal term birth and continuing throughout normal nursing. In contrast, in the guinea pig, sheep and monkey, the most active period of brain growth is before birth, whilst in species such as rat and rabbit the prominent period of brain growth is after birth. Other reasons for using the piglet are that the distribution of fatty acids in sow milk is very similar to that in human milk, and that the lipid composition of the pig brain is also very similar to that of the human.

The piglets were taken at birth, and studied after feeding the formula for 5, 10, 15 or 25 days; 25 days is the normal duration of suckling for this species. The control group of piglets was fed sow milk from birth. The formula fat was similar to that in many term infant formula and contained about 34% 18:2 n–6, and similar levels of 18:3 n–3 to sow or human milk (0.8%), but little of the long chain n–6 or n–3 fatty acids. The piglets were taken right after birth, and thus were colostrum-deprived. Pig immunoglobulins were prepared from pig blood and resuspended in the formulas to provide passive immunity. The animals were hand fed the formula every three hours round the clock for the first 72 hours of life, then later trained

Effects of current infant formula on brain and retinal lipid development

to feeders attached to the side of the pig cage, and fed every three hours. The sow milk fed pigs were left with their mothers to suckle normally. The fatty acids of the phospholipids from the whole brain synaptic terminal membranes and retina, as well as liver, plasma and red blood cells were studied. The analyses of the brain synaptic plasma membranes and retina showed that the percent 22:5 and 22:6 n–3 and the total n–3 fatty acids were higher in the sow milk fed piglets than in the piglets fed formula. In contrast to the n–3 fatty acids, the n–6 fatty acids 22:4 n–6 and 22:5 n–6 in the pig brain synaptic membranes and retina were higher than in the sow fed animals. *Figure 1* shows the results for phosphatidylethanolamine (EPG) in the synaptic membranes and retina. The levels of 20:4 n–6 in the brain and retina were not altered by the feeding of the formula. The difference between the group became significantly greater with increasingly duration of feeding, $p < 0.0001$. These data are illustrated for the synaptic plasma membrane EPG in *figure 2*.

Consideration of whole brain accretion as mg of fatty acid per whole brain, rather than percent fatty acid distributions of carbon chain 20 and 22 n–6 and n–3 fatty acids is clearly important to defining the limitation or adequacy of formula fats to support normal brain development. In the sow milk fed piglets, the absolute quantity of n–3 fatty acids in the brain increased from 5 to 25 days of age (*figure 3*). In the formula fed piglets on the other hand, the quantity of n–3 fatty acids in the brain

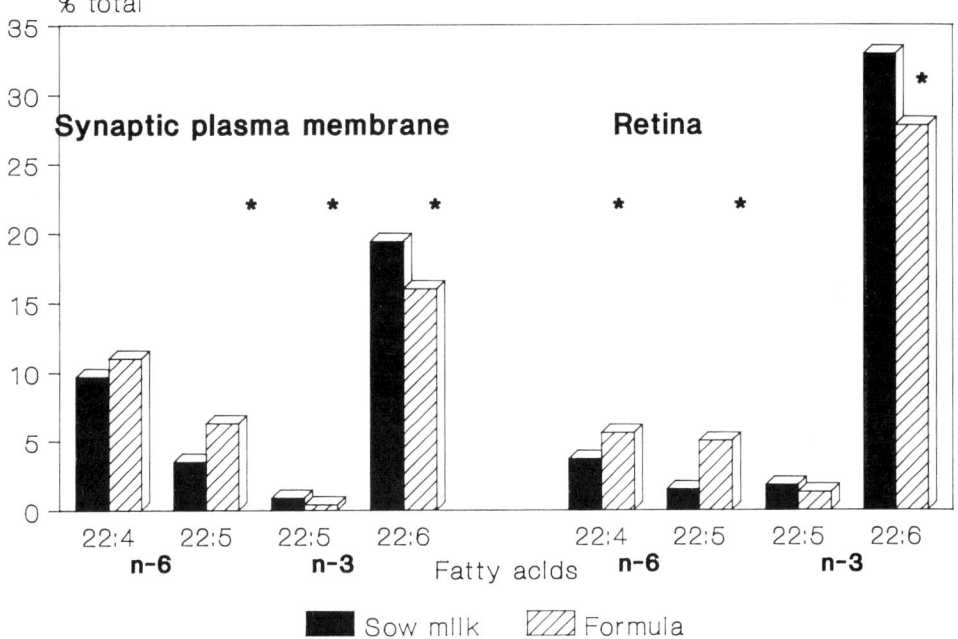

* $p<0.5$ formula compared to sow group

Figure 1. EPG n–6 and n–3 LCP.

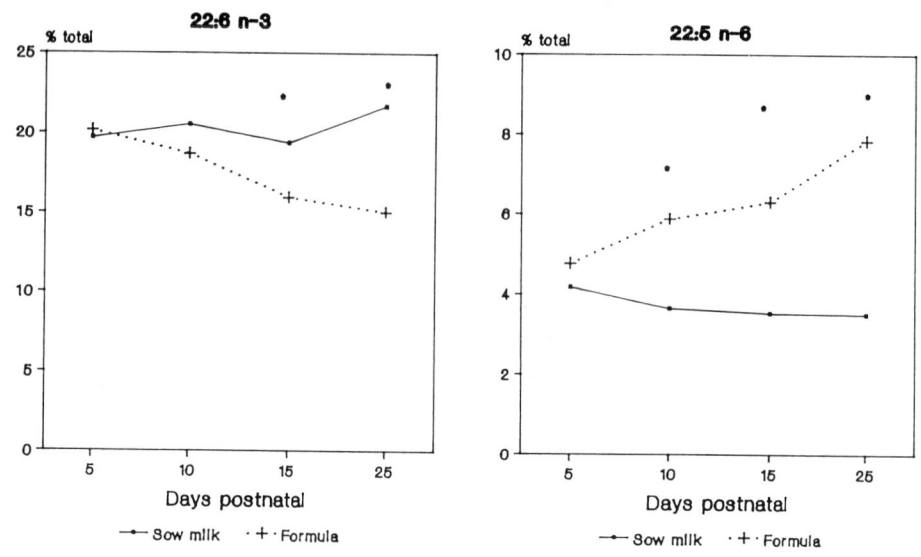

* p < 0.05 formula compared to milk grou

Figure 2. Synaptic plasma membrane EPG.

changed little with increasing age. The mg 20 and 22 carbon n–6 fatty acids per whole brain showed a small and fairly constant increase in the sow milk group to 25 days of age, but a substantial and significantly greater increase in the formula fed animals (figure 3). The total quantity of carbon chain 20 and 22 n–6 plus n–3 fatty acids in the whole brain showed an increase with increasing age, but no difference due to feed (figure 4). Specifically, the carbon chain 22 n–3 fatty acids increased from 83 ± 3.5 mg, per whole brain at 5 days of age to 136.7 ± 1.1 mg/brain at 25 days of age in the sow milk group, but was 80.8 ± 1.8 mg per at 5 days and only 89.6 ± 2.2 mg/brain 20 days later in the animals fed formula. These calculations show that once the brain has attained n–3 long chain polyenoic fatty acids, they are retained and do not, on a mass basis, decline. The carbon chain 22 n–6 fatty acids increased from 65.3 ± 1.8 mg per brain at 5 days of age to 114 ± 2.8 mg per brain at 25 days in the formula fed animals (figure 3). Thus, brain growth in the formula fed animals was accompanied by deposition of long chain n–6 fatty acids, rather than long chain n–3 fatty acids as normally occurs. The total carbon chain 22 n–6 plus n–3 fatty acids in the brain at 25 days of age was 216.8 ± 2.6 mg in the milk fed, and was similar at 204.9 ± 5.0 mg in the formula fed piglets (figure 4). The unsaturation index (calculated from the number of double bonds and the weight percent of each fatty acid) also was not altered by formula feeding. This constancy of total long chain polyenoic content was quite different to the effect of the formula in the liver. In liver, there was a significant difference in the total quantity of n–6 plus n–3 long chain polyenoics and a lower unsaturation index in the formula fed than in the sow-milk fed piglets. The analysis of the retinal phospholipid fatty acids

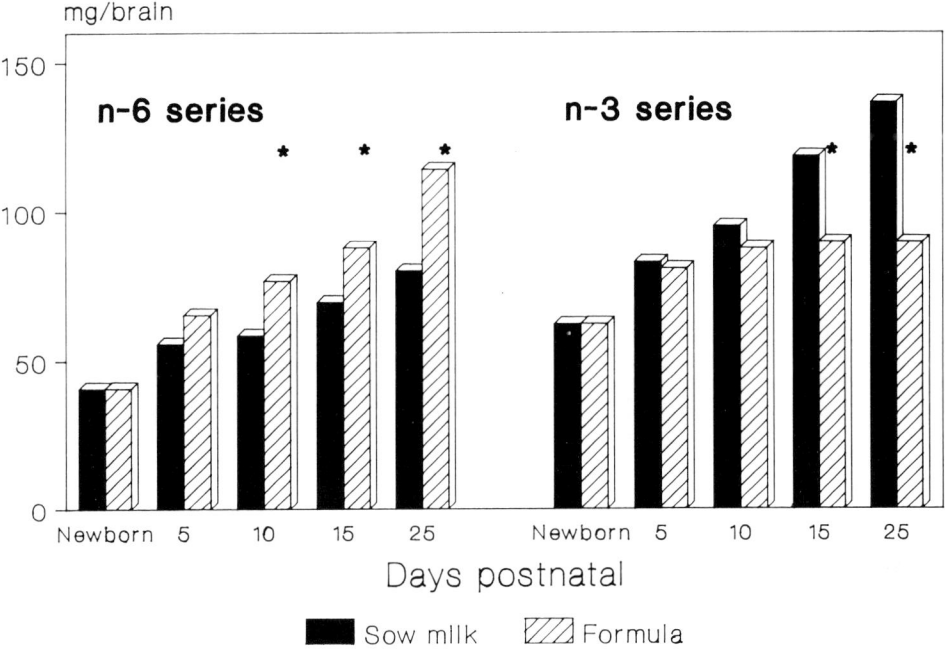

Figure 3. Brain carbon chain 22 LCP.

showed an identical pattern of increased n–6 polyenoics and decreased n–3 polyenoics in the formula group to that seen in the synaptic membranes.

Dr Clandinin has alluded to the comparative analyses of the effect of diet on fatty acids of brain, liver, plasma phospholipid and the red blood cell phosphatidylcholine and phosphatidylethanolamine. These analyses were done to answer the question as to whether or not it is valid to extrapolate from plasma and red cell membranes to what is happening in the brain and the liver of infants fed various formulas. The decrease in 22:6 n–3 in the brain, retina and liver of the animals fed formula was apparent in the analyses of their plasma phospholipid and red blood cell phosphatidylcholine and ethanolamine. In all cases the amount of 22:6 n–3 was significantly lower in the formula than in the milk fed group. If one looks at the n–6 series, however, the significant elevation of 22:4 n–6 and 22:5 n–6 seen in the brain, retina and liver ($p < 0.0001$) was not found in the analysis of the red cell phospholipids.

The conclusions of these studies in the piglet may be summarized as:

1. because the levels of the carbon chain n–6 fatty acids specifically 22:5 n–6 were increased in the brain of piglets fed formula with no long chain n–6 fatty acids, the desaturases, including the Δ-4 desaturase, must be active in the neonatal liver and/or brain;

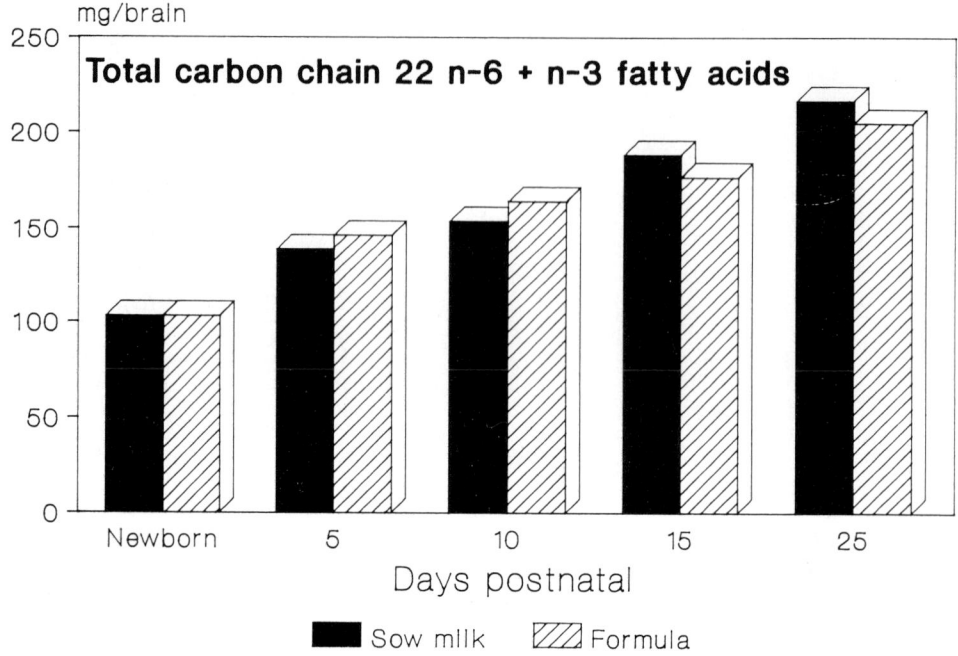

Formula and sow group similar, p> 0.5.

Figure 4. Brain carbon chain 22 LCP.

2. formula with less than 1% 18:3 n–3 leads to reduced brain carbon chain 20 and 22 n–3 fatty acid accretion. This could be due to competitive desaturation and/or acylation of n–3 fatty acids due to the high formula content of 18:2 n–6, or it could reflect a specific requirement for carbon chain 20 and 22 n–3, but not for n–6 fatty acids. Alternatively it could be explained by inadequate 18:3 n–3 in the formula;

3. the plasma and red blood cell fatty acids reflect depletion of the carbon chain 22 n–3 fatty acid in the brain and liver of the formula fed animal. They do not, however, predict organ desaturase activities or the increase in the n–6 series fatty acids.

Dr Carlson had published studies to demonstrate that preterm infants fed formulas have significantly lower levels of 22:6 n–3 in their red blood cell phosphatidylethanolamine than preterm infants fed breast milk. Because of the results of the effects of formula in the piglet, it seems possible that the low 22:6 n–3 levels in infants fed formula may be caused by something other than low desaturase enzyme activity. Comparative studies of β-oxidation of 18:2 n–6, 18:3 n–3 and other fatty acids have inferred that proportionately more dietary 18:3 n–3 undergoes oxidation than is the case for 18:2 n–6. Further, whereas dietary 18:3 n–3 is partitioned between oxidation and desaturation, dietary 22:6 n–3 is efficiently acylated into phospholipids. This suggests that formulas containing 1% or less fatty acids as 18:3 n–3 and no longer chain n–3 fatty acids may not provide adequate 18:3 n–3 to support optimal rates of 22:6 n–3 synthesis. The level of 18:3 n–3 in Enfamil-Premature® and Special Care® as published by Dr Carlson in 1986 was about 0.6 to 0.9% fatty acids. Human breast milk on the other hand contains about this amount of 18:3 n–3, but also contains significant quantities of longer chain n–3 fatty acids. Preterm breast milk collected in Vancouver typically contains about 0.9% 18:3 n–3 and 0.9% long chain polyenoics of the n–3 series, (about 34% Kcal 18:3 n–3 and 34% Kcal as longer chain n–3 polyenoic fatty acids), Table I. Considering the total quantity of n–3 fatty acids in breast milk and the greater biological activity of 22:6 n–3 than 18:3 n–3, it seems reasonable to predict that formula with less than 2% 18:3 n–3 may be deficient in n–3 fatty acids. Current preterm infant formulas containing soybean oil rather than corn oil contain 2% fatty acids (about 0.97% Kcal) as 18:3 n–3 (Table I). It was hypothesized that the higher amount of 18:3 n–3 in these formulas might limit or avoid the depletion of 22:6 n–3 in preterm infants fed formula. A study was, therefore, undertaken to determine the effect of feeding Special Care® with 2% 18:3 n–3 on the plasma and red cell phospholipids of low birth weight infants. The infants were appropriate for gestational age, of 950-1 250 g birth weight, and were studied from the day that of full oral feeds (designated as 120 ml per kg body weight per day) commenced for a further 28 days of full oral feeding. The infants were fed with: 1. their own mother's expressed breast milk; 2. Special Care® formula; or 3. mixed feeds of breast milk and formula. At the present time, most of the very premature infants in the nursery in Vancouver receive mixed feeds of formulas and milk. This is usually due to insufficient milk supply. The infants had a mean gestational age of 28 to 29 weeks at birth, and were an average of 12-13 days of age when they reached full oral feeding. Typically infants born at this stage of gestation require several days to weeks of parenteral nutrition during which the parenteral feeds first supply all, and then a progressively decreasing proportion of the nutrient intake as the infants are gradually weaned onto oral feeding. The range of postnatal age of the infants when full oral feeds commenced was 7 to 33 days of age. Thus, the postnatal age after 28 days of full feeding had been completed was 35 and up to 61 days.

Table I. N–6 and n–3 fatty acids of expressed breast milk and preterm infant formula

Fatty acids (% total)	Breast milk	Formula
18:2 n–6	11.1 ± 0.8	19.7
20:4 n–6	0.8 ± 0.1	–
22:4 n–6	0.2 ± 0.0	–
22:5 n–6	0.1 ± 0.0	–
18:3 n–3	0.9 ± 0.2	2.0
20:5 n–3	0.2 ± 0.0	–
22:5 n–3	0.2 ± 0.0	–
22:6 n–3	0.5 ± 0.1	–

The formula was Special Care®, Ross Laboratories, Columbus, Ohio – indicates less than 0.1% fatty acids. Adapted from Innis et al., Am J Clin Nutr 1990; 51:994-1000.

The n–6 and n–3 fatty acid levels in the plasma phospholipid and red blood cell phosphatidylcholine and ethanolamine after 28 days of feeding were similar among the infants irrespective of whether they were fed formula or breast milk (*Table II*). The only difference found was a higher level of 18:2 in the infants fed formula rather than breast milk. The level of 20:4 n–6, 22:4 n–6, and all of the n–3 fatty acids were similar among the infant groups. The total carbon chain 20 and 22 n–6 series, and the n–3 series and the ratio of 22:4 n–6 and 22:5 n–6 to 22:6 n–3 was also calculated in an attempt to detect any possible preferential desaturation of n–6 over n–3 fatty acids. The total long chain n–6, total long chain n–3 fatty acids, and the ratios between the two series were identical in the plasma red blood cell phosphatidylcholine and phosphatidylethanolamine among the infants. The conclusion from this study was that the plasma and red blood cell 2.0 20:4, 22:4 and 22:5 n–6, 20:5, 22:5 and 22:6 n–3 of low birth weight infants fed formula with about 20% 18:2 n–6 and 2% 18:3 are similar after 28 days of full oral feeding to that of infants fed breast milk.

The conclusions from the studies conducted in Vancouver can be summarized to suggest:

1. The requirements list of new born infants for 18:3 n–3 depends on the tissue reserves of carbon chain 20 and 22 n–3 fatty acids. Thus, based on the lower tissue reserves of the premature than term infant, as discussed by Dr Clandinin, it is reasonable to suggest that the 18:3 n–3 requirement is higher in a preterm infant than in a term infant.

2. The dietary 18:3 n–3 requirement will depend on the need for carbon chain 20 and 22 n–3 fatty acid synthesis. As a result, the dietary 18:3 n–3 requirement

Table II. Fatty acids of plasma phospholipid (PL) and red blood cell phosphatidylcholine (PC) and phosphatidylethanolamine (PE) of premature infants fed breast milk, formula or mixed feeds of breast milk and formula for 28 days

Tissue	Fatty acid (% total)					
Group	20:4 n–6	22:4 n–6	22:5 n–6	20:5 n–3	22:5 n–3	22:6 n–3
PL						
Breast milk	10.6 ± 0.7	0.6 ± 0.1	0.8 ± 0.2	0.5 ± 0.1	0.7 ± 0.1	2.8 ± 0.3
Formula	8.6 ± 0.5	0.5 ± 0.0	0.9 ± 0.1	0.7 ± 0.1	0.7 ± 0.0	2.4 ± 0.2
Mixed	8.0 ± 0.4	0.6 ± 0.1	0.9 ± 0.2	0.8 ± 0.1	0.7 ± 0.1	2.7 ± 0.2
PC						
Breast milk	6.9 ± 0.4	0.9 ± 0.3	0.6 ± 0.2	0.4 ± 0.1	0.6 ± 0.1	1.2 ± 0.1
Formula	5.9 ± 0.3	0.6 ± 0.1	0.6 ± 0.1	0.4 ± 0.0	0.5 ± 0.1	1.6 ± 0.3
Mixed	6.8 ± 0.8	0.6 ± 0.1	0.5 ± 0.1	0.5 ± 0.0	0.5 ± 0.1	1.6 ± 0.3
PE						
Breast milk	26.1 ± 0.9	6.4 ± 0.2	1.3 ± 0.2	0.8 ± 0.1	2.3 ± 0.1	7.0 ± 0.5
Formula	23.6 ± 0.8	6.6 ± 0.2	1.2 ± 0.1	0.9 ± 0.1	2.9 ± 0.2	6.1 ± 0.2
Mixed	24.8 ± 1.4	6.4 ± 0.5	1.2 ± 0.1	1.0 ± 0.1	2.4 ± 0.3	6.1 ± 0.6

There were no statistically significant ($p < 0.05$) differences among the groups in any of the fatty acids given. Adapted from Innis *et al.*, *Am J Clin Nutr* 1990; 51:994-1000.

in an infant fed formula will be higher than in an infant fed breast milk. This is because the infant fed formula must synthesize all of the needed long chain polyenoics, whereas an infant fed breast milk consumes preformed 22:6 n–3. Extending from this, formulas with similar levels of 18:3 n–3 to breast milk, but no 22:6 n–3 are likely to provide inadequate 18:3 n–3 to support the requirements of the formula.

3. Formula containing less than 1% 18:3 n–3 (about 0.4% Kcal), similar to human milk and no longer chain n–3 fatty acids lead to increased n–6 long chain polyenoic accretion and decreased 22:6 n–3 accretion in the growing brain. The importance of the quantity of 18:2 n–6 and the 18:2 n–6 to 18:3 n–3 ratio in the formula on long chain polyenoic synthesis, specifically that of 22:6 n–3, still requires further investigation.

Discussion

Chairman: I think we're ready for some questions here and it looks to me as if you have at least 6 or 7 minutes if we give you the 30 minutes as everyone else has done. Does anyone want to ask a question?

J.M. Bourre: I'm afraid maybe I missed two points in your talk because I don't understand why you can conclude that in fact the preterm infant fed formula needs higher amount of alpha-linolenic acid than the others.

S. Innis: I have suggested that the dietary requirement for 18:3 n–3 is dependent on whether or not the infant also ingests 22:6 n–3. If there is no dietary source of 22:6 n–3, the infant must synthesize it. Thus the dietary requirement for 18:3 n–3 should be higher than with a diet 22:6 n–3. So, in the situation of breast milk, the infant receives about 0.3% Kcal as preformed 22:6 n–3, and about 0.3-0.4% Kcal 18:3 n–3. In the infant fed formula, there is no dietary source of 22:6 n–3. The formula must provide sufficient 18:3 n–3 to allow for *in vivo* synthesis of an equivalent amount of 22:6 n–3 to that received in the diet of the breast milk fed infant. Because 18:3 n–3 is not converted on an equimolar basis to 22:6 n–3, that is much of it is oxidized, it is reasonable that 0.3-0.4% Kcal (about 1% fatty acids) 18:3 n–3 in formulas is too low. By increasing the 18:3 n–3 in the formula to three times that in breast milk we have found that the red blood cell 22:6 n–3 levels of the premature infants could be maintained for 28 days of full feeding.

C. Galli: Just two comments. Several years ago we found very similar results with the rat concerning the influences of different diets of n–3 and n–6 fatty acids and our conclusions were that brain polyunsaturates remain constant. Total desaturation also remains constant. So that given the different species, this phenomenon of maintenance of brain total polyunsaturates is a constant thing. My second point is that as you mentioned it is very difficult to compare the influence of diet on the profiles of plasma lipids and those of the tissues because different lipid classes in plasma may be differently affected by the diet. If you give high levels of EPA (20:5 n–3), you displace 20:4 n–6 from phospholipids. Going through the glycerides, you have a reduction in one phospholipid class and increase in another, so it's very difficult then to estimate changes in the tissues. This requires further studies.

Chairman: I have two further minor questions for Dr Innis. As you know I have shown different findings than you have with lower linolenic. On the data that I'm going to show you tomorrow we're feeding actually higher linolenic acid levels and while after 28 days the difference is not so marked, over the first 5 or 6 months it becomes very different. I would agree with you that the higher linolenic is supporting the red blood cell 22:6 n–3 for some period of time, but it's not supporting it beyond the first three or four weeks. As I look at your data and mine I was trying to find out what may be different in our studies. One of the things that strikes me when I look at your data is the high level of 22:6 n–3 in the milk of your mothers and the relatively low 18:2 n–6 compared to US mothers' milk. I think you've got the mention Canadians do not eat as much 18:2 n–6 as in the States. I'm wondering first of all if you think that the status of mother was important.

S. Innis: Do you mean the babies in Vancouver were born with a better 22:6 n–3 status?

Chairman: I mean that you'd like to think that when they were born 3 months early. The other question I would have is: did any of your formula fed babies receive human milk?

S. Innis: No. Babies who were fed both formula and breast milk were assigned to the mixed fed group.

Chairman: Is this a pure dietary group?

S. Innis: Yes, that's why the infants were split into three diet groups. The formula fed babies received formula only, the breast milk babies received only breast milk, and the mixed group received mixed feeds.

Chairman: So none of them received human milk before they were on this diet?

S. Innis: No, very little. Diet records were kept from birth, right through the study. I think you've alluded to a very important point with regard to preterm infants. It is important that the results from these studies do not give the impression that preterm infants are doing well in regards to their 22:6 n–3 status. When these infants are compared to term infants (*figure 5*) at the start of full oral feeds, the premature infants have lower levels of 22:6 n–3 in their plasma phospholipid and red blood cell phosphatidylcholine and phosphatidylethanolamine than do term infants. *Figure 5* illustrates the level of 22:6 n–3 in the red blood cell phosphatidylethanolamine of term and preterm infants at birth and at 3 days of age, and in term infants fed breast milk for 28 days, and the premature infants at the start of full oral feeding and after 28 days feeding with breast milk. Although the levels of 22:6 n–3 in the premature infants were maintained by 28 days feeding with formula, the levels in these infants are lower than in normal term babies or that present in preterm babies

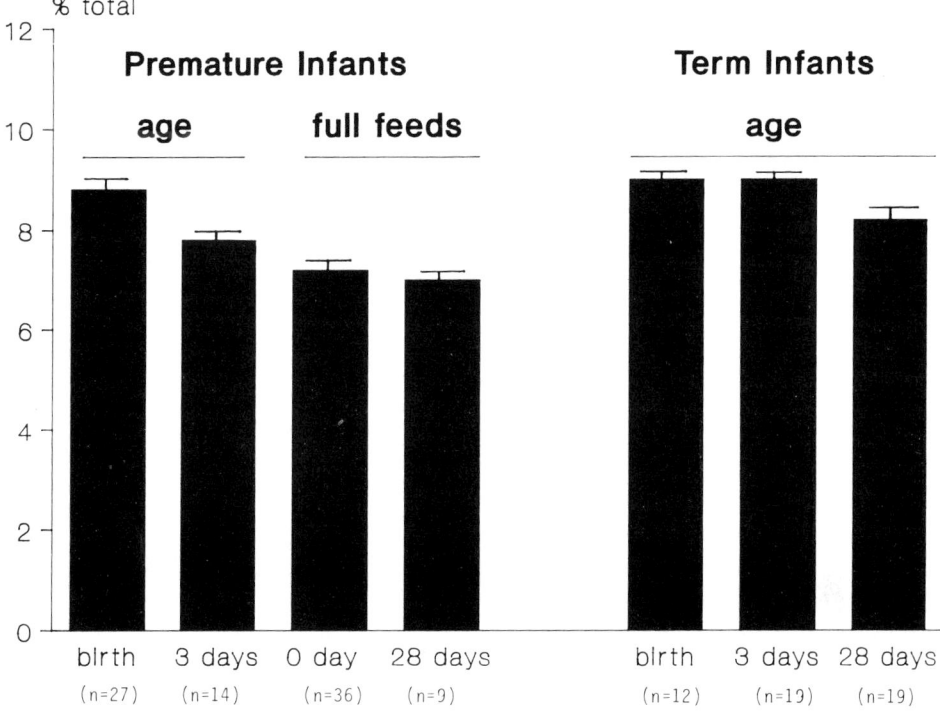

Figure 5. Red blood cell EPG 22:6 n–3. 28 days feeding was with the mother's breast milk for both the premature and term infants. 0 day full feeds (120 ml/kg/day) was at 7 to 33 days postnatal. The data are mean values ± SEM. The decline from birth to 3 days postnatal, and from 3 days postnatal to 0 the start of full feeds (0 day) was significant ($p < 0.05$). There was no statistically significant difference during 28 days of feeding with breast milk in either the term or preterm infants.

at birth. When Dr Carlson discusses the work she's been doing on visual acuity, and whether or not we can improve the 22:6 n–3 levels in very premature babies, my opinion is that there is a substantial problem with the 22:6 n–3 status of all of these infants, irrespective of whether they are fed breast milk or current formulas. All these infants have lower 22:6 n–3 level than term babies. In a recent study of the impact of early nutritional support on 92 preterm infants of about 28 weeks gestation, followed for up to 35 days of parenteral feeding, we found that the level of 22:6 n–3 in the red blood cell decreased with increasing time on parenteral nutrition. The levels of 22:6 n–3 were similar in cord blood, red blood cells and plasma of babies born at 20 to 41 weeks of gestation. This suggests that a very important possible difference among results from different centres is likely to relate to how aggressive the neonatologist is in getting the babies onto oral feeds. The longer the delay in achieving full oral feeds, the more depleted the babies become in 22:6 n–3. The results generated in our nursery show that the depletion of 22:6 n–3 is not improved by either breast milk or current formulas. The "depleted" level of 22:6

n–3, however, is maintained without further significant decrease by feeding breast milk.

Chairman: I think that is a good point because you apparently helped your population of babies whereas we can't get our babies on full feed as early.

S. Innis: The mean postnatal age for our babies was 12 days; about a week faster than you have reported.

Chairman: I think that it's a very good point. There are differences in units and different managements and we have also seen there is a very high inverse correlation between postnatal age 22:6 n–3 in the red blood cell. It has nothing to do with gestational age.

B. Koletzko: I must admit I was rather surprised by your results because a number of studies in young adults show that feeding alpha-linolenic acid does not increase n–3 FA and partly because of our own observations which probably do not allow this confusion and I have some concerns of the same sort that Sue Carlson raised. I wonder whether there were other works which have compared breast fed infants and formula fed infants and of the effect of differences in alpha-linoleic to linoleic acid ratios. So I want to know whether you would agree whether one would need another group, maybe with the same linoleic acid and alpha-linolenic acid intake.

S. Innis: Are you alluding to the problem of ratios 18:2 to 18:3?

B. Koletzko: That's part of the question, I mean there's maybe a number of differences between the breast fed and formula fed infants other than just linoleic and alpha-linolenic acid.

S. Innis: Another possible difference is lipoprotein transport. Cholesterol levels are quite different between the formula fed and the breast fed infant. Whether or not there is any interaction with 22:6 n–3 status is unclear.

B. Koletzko: The other question I have is whether some of the infants or all of the infants got intravenous lipids.

S. Innis: Yes they did. The intake of IV lipid was identical among the groups. The total quantity of IV lipid received and the duration post IV lipid intake that the first blood sample was taken was recorded. During the 28 days study period that the babies were followed, all IV support had ceased, so the babies had at least 120 mL of formula or breast milk per kg per day. At the first blood sample there was no parenteral support; the time elapsed since the last IV lipid administration was about 46 hours. The total quantity of IV lipid received in the early postnatal period was identical in the breast milk and formula fed babies.

B. Koletzko: That was soybean emulsion?

S. Innis: It is the soybean oil emulsion, yes. Whether or not Dr Carlson's unit uses soybean rather than safflower, I am unsure.

Chairman: So do we. We have looked at this, but it cannot be done as a simple difference between groups with mean values. A repression analysis is needed because as Dr Innis pointed out, the babies varying in age over a whole month and clearly the older ones probably got more intravenous lipid than the younger ones.

B. Koletzko: Another question. You mentioned your possible inhibition of $\Delta 6$-desaturase by high linoleic acid. It's quite unusual in biochemistry to have such an inhibition, I just wondered whether you have some comments on possible mechanisms?

S. Innis: I am not sure that 55% or so 18:2 n–6 in the diet (intravenous) fat can be considered physiologically normal.

5

Essential fatty acid interconversion during the perinatal period. Influence of dietary factors

G. BÉRÉZIAT, G. THOMAS, P. CARDOT*, J. CHAMBAZ

Laboratoire de Biochimie, URA CNRS 1283, Faculté de Médecine Saint-Antoine, 27, rue Chaligny, 75571 Paris Cedex 12, France
* Département de Nutrition Humaine, INRA-Theix, Clermont-Ferrand, France

The importance of essential fatty acid has been related to their structural action, their specific interaction with membrane proteins or their ability to serve as precursors of lipid mediators. These compounds are autacoids, named also eicosanoids, which are the products of cyclooxygenase (prostaglandins, thromboxanes), of 5-lipoxygenase (leucotrienes) and of 12- or 15-lipoxygenases (other hydroperoxidized fatty acids) [1]. They interact with hormonal or other transducing mechanisms. Prostaglandins stimulate or inhibit adenylate-cyclase, leucotrienes and thromboxane stimulate the phospholipase specific of phosphatidylinositol diphosphate [2]. It has been recently reported that leucotrienes or other hydroxylated fatty acids might activate ion channels [3]. Their actions alter the ways by which cytoplasmic concentrations of second messengers (cyclic AMP, inositol triphosphate, calcium ion and diglycerides) are increased or decreased (*figure 1*). The messengers, in turn, alter the activity of various protein-kinases whom relevance for the regulation of enzyme activity and gene expression is well established.

The fatty acid precursors of eicosanoids are synthesized through elongation and desaturation processes which transform mainly linoleic acid into arachidonic acid and αlinolenic acid into eicosapentaenoic acid and docosahexaenoic acid [4,5] (*figure 2*). In order to understand the respective role of foetal liver, maternal liver and placenta for the supply of arachidonic acid to the foetus, we assayed Δ6- and Δ5-desaturase activities, elongase activity and fatty acyl CoA synthetase activities [6,7].

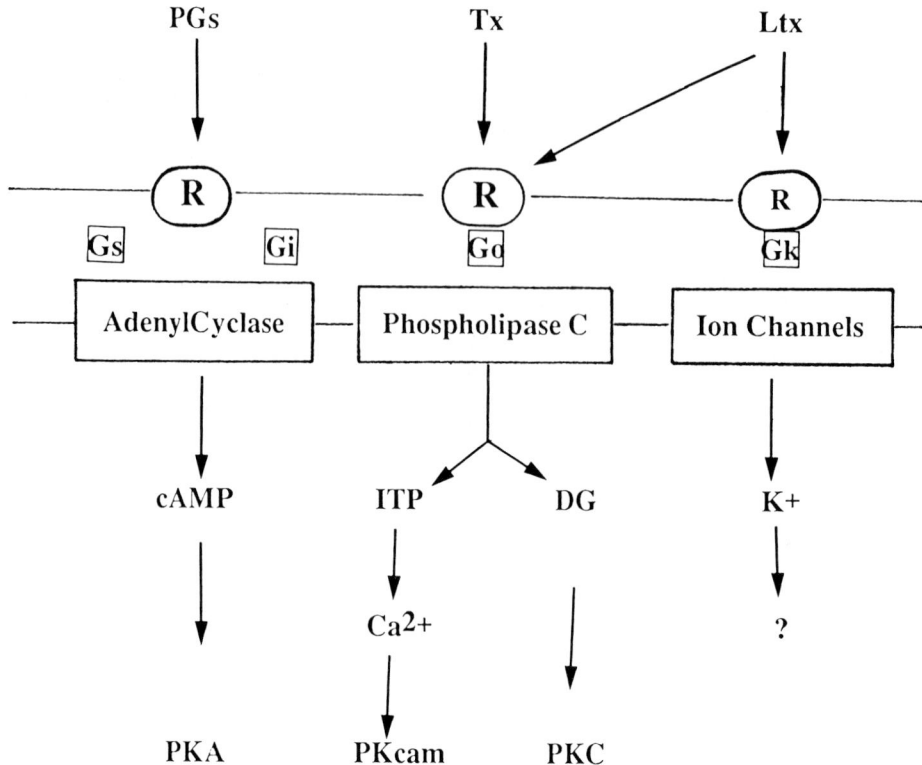

Figure 1. Transducing pathways for lipid mediators. PGs: prostaglandins; Tx: thromboxane; Ltx: leucotrienes; Gs, i, o, k: various GTP binding proteins; cAMP: cyclic adenosyl monophosphate; ITP: inositol triphosphate; DG: diacyl glycerol; PKA: protein-kinase A; PKcam: calmodulin-stimulated protein kinase; PKC: protein kinase C; R: receptor.

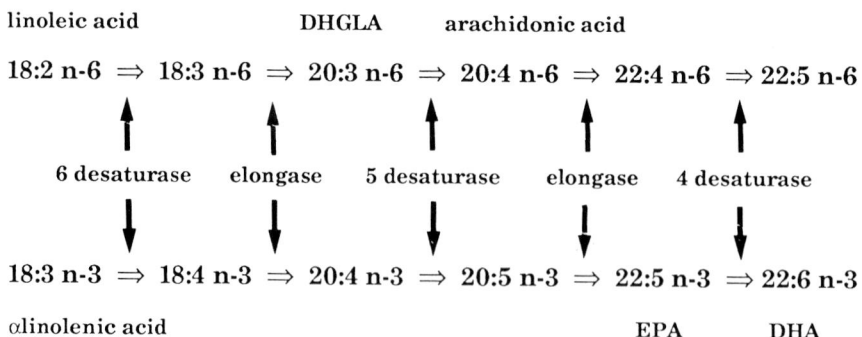

Figure 2. Linoleic and α interconversion pathways.

We first evidenced that both maternal and foetal liver microsomes desaturate at nearly the same rate linoleic acid into γlinolenic acid. There was no significant variation between day 19, 21 and 22 of the gestation. The Δ5-desaturase activity of maternal liver microsomes increases until day 21 of gestation and decreases after. This may be related to an increase of an inhibitory factor. Conversely, Δ5-desaturase activity of the foetal liver still increases at day 22, just before birth (*Table I*). Neither Δ6- nor Δ5-desaturase activity is found in placenta microsomes after day 15, 19 and 22 of pregnancy.

Table I. Δ 5-desaturase activities in rat and foetal liver

	Non-pregnant	Days of pregnancy		
		19th	21st	22nd
Rat liver	270 ± 44	302 ± 62	433 ± 105	112 ± 22
Foetal liver		58 ± 8	nd	150 ± 20

20:3 n–6 CoA 50μMol; results in pmol/min/mg microsomal protein.

The differences that we observed in the desaturation rates cannot be explained by variations of fatty acyl CoA synthetase activities which were always higher than desaturase activities in the different tissues tested. There was no significant difference between linoleic acid and dihomogammalinolenic acid activation. Pregnancy increases the activation of both fatty acids in the maternal liver but there was no variation according to the gestational age in either maternal liver, foetal liver or placenta.

The elongation process was monitored by malonyl CoA incorporation into γlinolenic acid. Its rate was two fold higher than Δ6-desaturase activity in control liver and maternal liver, and it remained constant during the pregnancy (*Table II*). As a consequence, elongation process cannot be considered as the limiting step in essential fatty acid interconversion in the maternal liver. In the foetus, the elongation rate was lower than Δ6- or Δ5-desaturase activities. Since γlinolenic acid does not accumulate in foetal lipids, this suggests that foetal liver plays a minor role in arachidonic acid supply to the growing foetus, the rate of the biosynthetic pathway being necessarily slow.

Table II. γlinoleic acid elongation process in placenta and maternal or foetal liver (pmol/min/mg microsomal protein)

Control liver	310 ± 31
Liver from pregnant rats at day 19	325 ± 14
Liver from pregnant rats at day 22	317 ± 53
Placenta	not detected
Foetal liver at day 19	99 ± 16
Foetal liver at day 22	135 ± 15

Furthermore, if we compare arachidonic acid production rate by foetal liver, maternal liver and placenta, we can establish that maternal liver plays a major role even at the terminal steps of the gestational process. It produces 100 fold more arachidonic acid than foetal liver at day 22 (*Table III*). This can explain arachidonic acid decreases in plasma lipids of the foetus just after the birth [8]. The existence of an essential fatty acid gradient between the mother and the foetus suggests that placenta plays an important role for arachidonic acid transfer to the foetus since it accumulates this fatty acid as compared to maternal plasma lipids. But it is devoid of any desaturase activity by itself.

Table III. Comparative arachidonic acid synthesis by placenta, maternal or foetal liver

	Total arachidonic acids synthesis	
	Total organ weight (g)	20:4 production (mol/min)
Foetal liver		
day 15	0.004 ± 0.001	ND
day 19	0.110 ± 0.014	0.03 ± 0.01
day 22	0.255 ± 0.25	0.25 ± 0.09
Placenta		
day 22	0.36 ± 0.08	ND
Maternal liver		
day 22	11.5 ± 1.6	21.9 ± 5.0

In order to examine if the nutritional requirement of essential fatty acid during pregnancy might favour essential fatty acid deficiency, we fed pregnant rats and control rats on saturated fat diet or corn oil diet [9]. We have also examined the effect of sucrose versus glucose as dietary carbohydrate since we previously demonstrated that sucrose accelerated essential fatty acid deficiency in weanling rat (*figures 3 and 4*). The pregnant rats fed on saturated diet and their foetuses exhibited a strong decrease in linoleic acid as non-pregnant rats, irrespective of the carbohydrate diet. The arachidonic acid content of plasma and microsomal liver lipids did not decrease in control rats fed 3 weeks with saturated fat. In pregnant rats and their foetuses, the decrease in arachidonic acid content of plasma and liver lipids was more obvious when sucrose was the carbohydrate instead of glucose.

This difference reflects altered modifications of the desaturase activities in essential fatty acid deprived sucrose-fed rats as respect to essential fatty acid deprived glucose-fed rats. The essential fatty acid deprivation strongly stimulates Δ6-desaturase activity in both control and pregnant glucose-fed rats (*figure 5*). There was no modification in sucrose-fed control rats and only a slight increase in pregnant sucrose-fed rats. But in sucrose-fed rats, the essential fatty acid deprivation slows down the increase of Δ5-desaturase activity observed at day 21 of gestation. The Δ5-desaturase activity remains very high in glucose-fed rats at that gestational stage (*figure 6*).

Essential fatty acid interconversion during the perinatal period

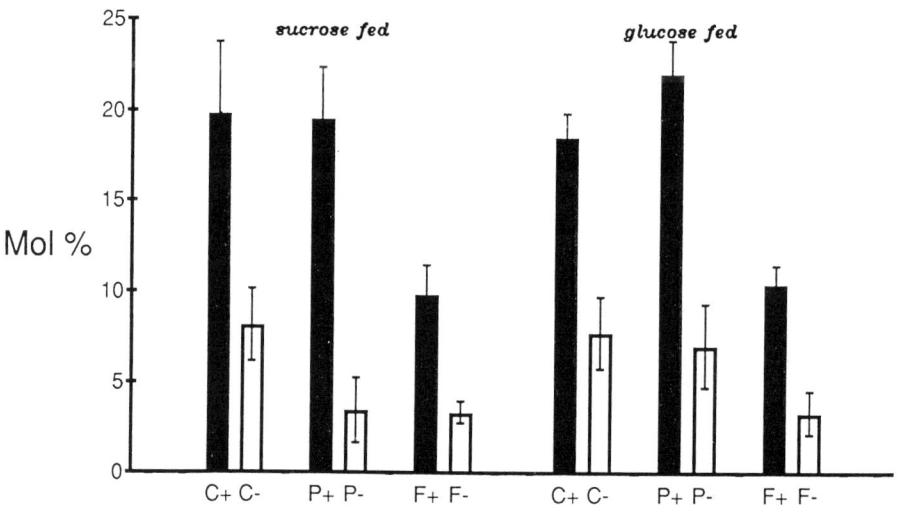

Figure 3. Linoleic acid status of plasma lipids in sucrose or glucose fed rats during essential fatty acid deficiency. C: control rat, P: pregnant rat; F: foetus; +: corn oil fed rat; −: saturated fat fed rats.

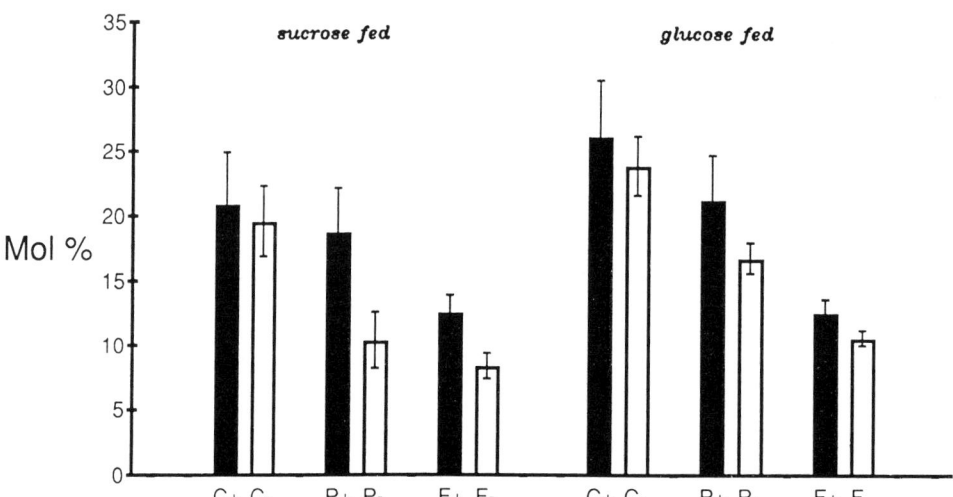

Figure 4. Arachidonic acid status of plasma lipids in sucrose or glucose fed rats during essential fatty acid deficiency. Symbols as in figure 3.

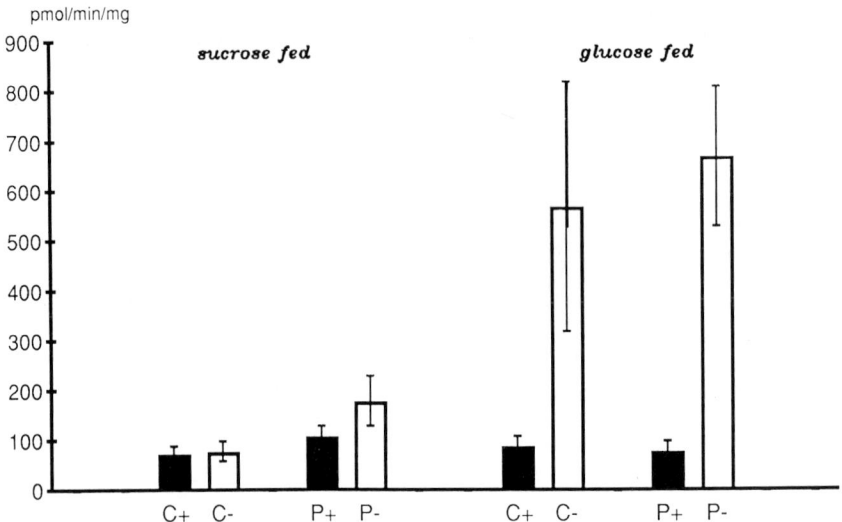

Figure 5. Δ6-desaturase activity in rat liver; effect of sucrose versus glucose and effect of essential fatty acid deficiency symbols as in figure 3.

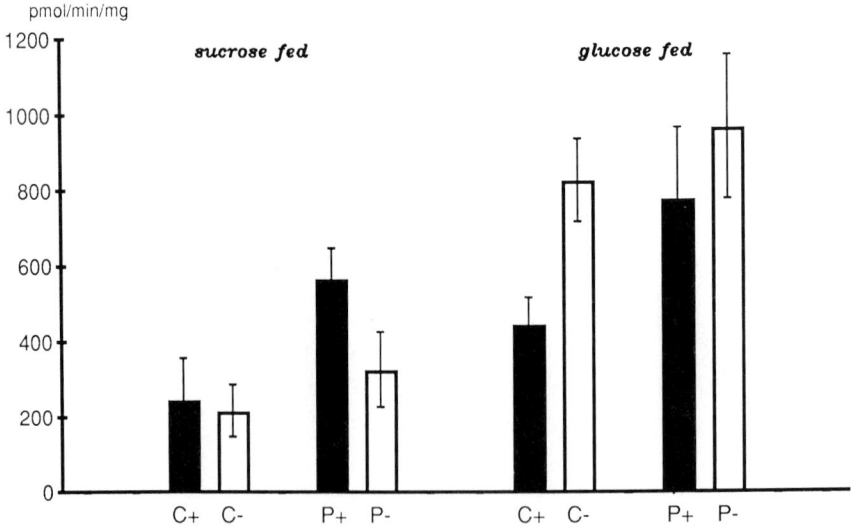

Figure 6. Δ6-desaturase activity in rat liver; effect of sucrose versus glucose and effect of essential fatty acid deficiency symbols as in figure 3.

From these experiments we suggest that both Δ5- and Δ6-desaturase activities are under the control of nutritional and hormonal factors as already suggested [10, 11]. The way this control is carried out remains to be established and better understanding of this regulation needs elucidation of protein and gene structure.

The molecular cloning of Δ9-desaturase in rat liver and mouse adipocytes has been achieved last year [12]. The 5' flanking region of the gene has been examined and tested as chimeric construct with the chloramphenicol acetyl transferase gene. In addition to the classical TATA box for polymerase binding and to GC box for SP1 fixation, several regulatory elements have been described (*figure 7*). These are glucocorticoids- and cyclic AMP-responsive elements and a fat specific element which are implicated in adipocyte differentiation. Such elements might also be implicated in the Δ6- and Δ5-desaturase gene induction by glucose and essential fatty acid deprivation. Variation in estrogene secretion during pregnancy might induce some effects through Estradiol responsive elements. Such elements have been described in the flanking region of apolipoprotein E gene [13].

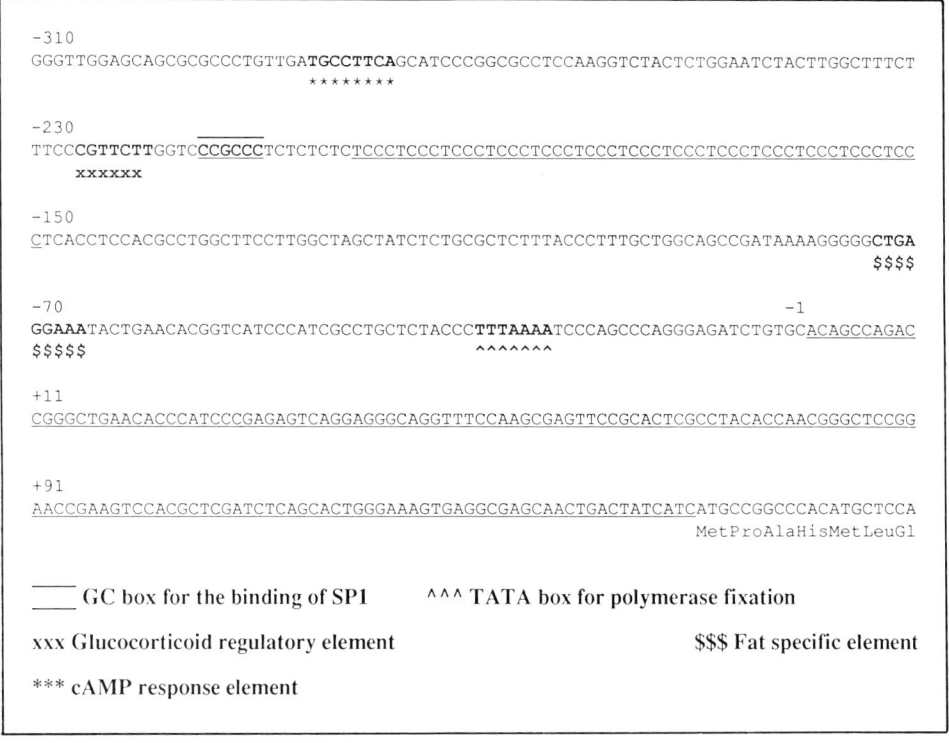

Figure 7. The promoter region of the 5' and of fatty acid synthetase gene.

Conclusion

– Foetal liver desaturase activity cannot account for the supply of arachidonic acid to the foetus.
– Placenta microsomes are not able to convert linoleic acid into arachidonic acid. But placenta can accumulate arachidonic acid in order to transfer it to the foetus.
– Pregnancy is a critical period for essential fatty acid deficiency.
– The liver counteracts essential fatty acid deficiency by a rapid adjustment of desaturase activities.
– Sucrose favours the onset of essential fatty acid deficiency by repressing Δ6-desaturase activities.
– To understand better the regulation of essential fatty acid interconversion, cloning of Δ6-, Δ5- and Δ4-desaturase genes is required.
– The 5' flanking region of these genes might contain regulatory elements for nutritional and hormonal factors.

References

1. Needleman P., Turk G., Jakschik B.A., Morrisson A.R., Lefkowith J.B. (1986) *Ann Rev Biochem* 55:69-102.
2. Béréziat G. (1989) Prostaglandins. In: Curtis Prior P.B., ed. Biology and chemistry of prostaglandins and related eicosanoïds. Churchill-Livingstone, 198-201.
3. Kurashi Y., Ito H., Sugito T. *et al.* (1989) *Nature* 377:555-60.
4. Brenner R.R. (1974) *Mol Cell Biochem* 3:41-50.
5. Ayala S., Graviela G., Brenner R.R., Pelluffo R.O., Kunau W. (1973) *J Lipid Res* 14:296-301.
6. Chambaz J., Ravel D., Manier M.C., Pépin D., Mulliez N., Béréziat G. (1985) *Biol Neonate* 47:136-40.
7. Ravel D., Chambaz J., Pepin D., Manier M.C., Béréziat G. (1985) *Biochim Biophys Acta* 833:161-4.
8. Satomi S., Matsuda I. (1973) *Biol Neonate* 22:1-8.
9. Cardot P., Chambaz J., Thomas G., Raissiguier Y., Béréziat G. (1987). *J Nutr* 117:1504-13.
10. Pelluffo R.O., Gomez-Dumm I.N.T., Dealaniz M.J.T., Brenner R.R. (1971) *J Nutr* 101:1075-84.
11. Gomez-Dumm I.N.T., De Analiz M.J.T., Brenner R.R. (1975) *J Lipid Res* 16:264-8.
12. Ntambi J.M., Buhrow S.A., Kaestner K.H., Christy R.J., Sibley E., Kelly T.J., Lane M.D. (1988) *J Biol Chem* 263:17291-300.
13. Smith J.D., Melian A., Leff T., Breslow J.L. (1988) *J Biol Chem* 263: 8300-8.

trates and you have a dilution factor with the linoleic acid given in the microsomes. The apparent specific activity is considerably affected by the amount of molecule you have in your system. The calculation of the rates of conversion is modified by these experimental conditions.

G. Béréziat: Yes, in some experiments we do the study with linoleic CoA and not with linoleic acid and ATP; we observe the same results. Of course the problem is to have a better model to look at the desaturation process, unfortunately as you know hepatocytes in primary cultures were very difficult to examine for the desaturation process. Of course there are some pitfalls and it might explain why we have a very high difference from an experiment to another experiment.

Chairman: Thank you very much.

SESSION III

Chairman: David HULL (United Kingdom)

6

Role of the placenta in the foetus fatty acids supply

V. CHIROUZE

*IMEDEX, Z.I. des Troques, BP 38,
69630 Chaponost, France*

I want, first, to thank the Doctors Ghisolfi and Putet and the Milupa Company for giving me the opportunity to participate in this workshop. As everybody knows here, normal growth of infants is dependent on an adequate supply of essential fatty acids. Like the adult the human foetus is unable to synthesize the essential fatty acid precursors which must then be supplied by the mother through the placenta. During pregnancy the concentration of polyenoic fatty acids increases in the foetus. Several studies tried to provide answers to the controversy concerning this essential fatty acid collection (*figure 1*).

First, accumulation of essential fatty acid in the foetus may result from an increased activity of the foeto-maternal unit by a preferential transfer of these fatty acids in later gestation. Second, enzymatic activity in the placenta may be responsible for the desaturation and elongation of these essential fatty acids. Third, after transfer of the fundamental fatty acids from the mother through the placenta, the foetus could metabolize these essential fatty acids.

Merieux Institute collects human placenta throughout the world in order to isolate placental blood from which various proteins such as albumin or immune globulins are extracted. Up to now blood-free placental tissue is not valorized when its lipids contain polyunsaturated fatty acids. The purpose of the work I will present now is to compare the lipid composition of placenta before and after blood extraction.

In both cases lipids are extracted with methanol/chloroform at room temperature in the presence of BHT as an antioxidant, according to the method of Folch. Determinations of phosphorous free, cholesterol and esterified cholesterol are performed directly on the whole lipid extract. The concentration of both triglycerides and free fatty acids are determined after separation by thin layer chromatography. These two fractions are then determined by internal standardization in gas liquid chromatogra-

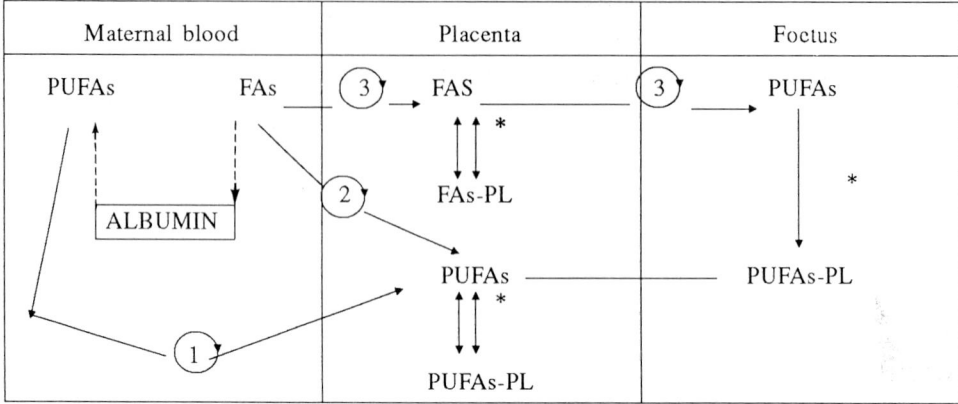

Figure 1. Mechanism of accumulation of EFAs in the foetus. *Esterification of fatty acids in the phospholipids.

phy. The fatty acid composition of total lipid extract and of the various lipid fractions are achieved by gas liquid chromatography and before the various lipid fractions are isolated by TLC and the appropriate areas of silica gel are scraped from the plate and submitted to the preparation of methyl ester derivatives. Finally, the determination of individual phospholipids is achieved by two-dimensional TLC. After separation of the various phospholipids on the silica gel plate the spots are scraped and submitted to phosphorous determination.

Concerning lipid content of both initial placenta and residual tissue, the results being expressed as mean values and standard deviations for N determinations, we noted that initial placenta seems to contain less total lipids than placental tissue, with reference to the same weight of tissue (*Table I*). This is quite normal because

Table I. Lipid composition of initial placenta and placental tissue

Lipid fractions	Placental tissue (N = 4)		Initial placenta (N = 3)	
	mg/100 g of tissue	% of total lipids	mg/100 g of tissue	% of total lipids
Phospholipids	1 289 ± 114	61,5 ± 5,4	501 ± 11	62,4 ± 1,4
Free fatty acids	285 ± 52	13,6 ± 2,5	146 ± 8	18,2 ± 1,0
Free cholesterol	341 ± 77	16,3 ± 3,7	148 ± 10	18,4 ± 1,2
Esterified cholesterol	34 ± 28	1,6 ± 1,0	8 ± 3,0	1 ± 0,4
Triglycerides	31 ± 6,0	1,5 ± 0,3	ND*	ND*
Ethylesters	115 ± 18	5,5 ± 0,8	–	–
Total lipids	2 095	100	803	100

* Not determined

placental blood, which contains less lipids than placental tissue, itself is still present in initial placenta. With regard to the total lipid composition of these two samples the only significant difference is the presence of ethyl esters in the placental tissue.

These esters are artefacts of the industrial process which uses ethanol to extract the placental blood. This explains also the smaller amount of free fatty acids found in this fraction. The proportions of the other lipid fractions were about the same in the initial and residual tissues. Phospholipids are the main components of these two fractions. We can see that phospholipids represent more than 60% of the total lipid extracts. Standard deviations show no significant difference from one industrial preparation to another; this indicates that this lipid composition is representative of the placental tissue industrially prepared.

When we compare the phospholipid distribution of these two samples, we observe a larger amount of lyso phosphatidyl ethanolamine in the placental tissue which might suggest a slight hydrolysis of the diacyl phosphatidyl ethanolamine during industrial process of blood extraction (*Table II*). The major components of the phospholipid fractions are phosphatidyl choline (about 40% of total phospholipid in placental tissue and about 30% in initial placenta), sphingomyelin (about 25% in the two samples) and phosphatidyl ethanolamine (about 18% in placental tissue and 32% in initial placenta).

Table II. Individual phospholipids distribution

Phospholipids	Moles % of total phospholipids	
	Placental tissue	Initial placenta
Phosphatidyl choline (PC)	40,8 ± 3,3	30,1 ± 1,2
Phosphatidyl ethanolamine (PE)	17,8 ±3,3	32 ± 1,0
Lyso PC	2,1 ± 0,3	0,7 ± 0,3
Lyso PE	7,1 ± 0,8	2,9 ± 0,5
Phosphatidyl inositol	2,9 ± 0,6	3,1 ± 0,7
Phosphatidyl serine	4,4 ± 0,5	7,6 ± 0,7
Sphingomyelin	25,1 ± 3,1	23,6 ± 1,6

The various lipid fractions (total lipids, phospholipids and free fatty acids) present a similar fatty acid composition (*Tables III and IV*). Both phospholipids and free fatty acids contain a high level of polyunsaturated fatty acids, with about 20% of arachidonic acid and about 3% of docosahexanoic acid. We observed no significant difference in the amount of polyunsaturated fatty acids between the two placental tissues, initial and residual. These results show that the blood extraction doesn't produce any fatty acid oxidation and that the placental tissue may represent a good source of polyunsaturated fatty acids.

We try to estimate the amount of fatty acids accumulated in one placenta during the pregnancy:
— one placenta weighs around 600 grams;
— after blood elimination, the residual tissue weighs around 200 grams;

Table III. Fatty acid composition of lipid fractions in initial placenta

Fatty acid	Total lipids	Phospholipids	Free fatty acids
15:0	0,3 ± 0,02	0,3 ± 0,01	0,2 ± 0,05
16:0	23,0 ± 0,2	27,9 ± 0,9	17,4 ± 0,4
16:1 N-7	2,9 ± 0,3	2,4 ± 0,3	3,1 ± 0,4
17:0	0,4 ± 0,01		–
18:0	11,8 ± 0,1	17,0 ± 0,6	9,7 ± 0,06
18:1 (N-9) + (N-7)	15,9 ± 0,02	17,0 ± 0,6	9,7 ± 0,06
18:2 N-6	12,1 ± 0,1	7,7 ± 0,04	13,2 ± 0,1
20:2 N-6	0,6 ± 0,01	0,5 ± 0,01	0,6 ± 0,03
20:3 N-6	4,6 ± 0,1	3,8 ± 0,05	6,4 ± 0,1
20:4 N-6	20,6 ± 0,1	18,7 ± 0,1	27,8 ± 0,4
22:4 N-6	1,8 ± 0,1	2,3 ± 0,07	1,2 ± 0,1
22:5 N-6	1,1 ± 0,02	1,2 ± 0,06	1,1 ± 0,1
22:5 N-3	0,7 ± 0,02	0,6 ± 0,1	0,3 ± 0,03
22:6 N-3	2,7 ± 0,6	3,0 ± 0,1	2,8 ± 0,2

Table IV. Fatty acid composition of lipid fractions in placental tissue

Fatty acid	Total lipids	Phospholipids	Free fatty acids
15:0	0,5 ± 0,1	0,3 ± 0,05	0,3 ± 0,1
16:0	23,6 ± 1,4	26,3 ± 1,8	20,3 ± 2,4
16:1 N-7	3,2 ± 0,5	2,2 ± 0,3	2,5 ± 0,5
17:0	0,7 ± 0,2	0,4 ± 0,1	0,3 ± 0,1
18:0	11,2 ± 0,7	16,1 ± 1,0	13,0 ± 0,9
18:1 (N-9) + (N-7)	14,8 ± 1,0	13,2 ± 1,1	18,8 ± 1,0
18:2 N-6	11,2 ± 1,2	8,9 ± 0,7	11,0 ± 1,1
20:2 N-6	0,8 ± 0,2	0,6 ± 0,2	0,6 ± 0,1
20:3 N-6	4,4 ± 0,4	3,3 ± 0,3	6,1 ± 0,9
20:4 N-6	19,6 ± 1,7	17,1 ± 1,2	20,1 ± 2,0
22:4 N-6	1,5 ± 0,3	1,6 ± 0,6	1,3 ± 0,4
22:5 N-6	1,0 ± 0,32	0,9 ± 0,3	1,3 ± 0,4
22:5 N-3	0,8 ± 0,2	0,7 ± 0,2	0,5 ± 0,2
22:6 N-3	3,2 ± 0,9	2,6 ± 0,7	3,4 ± 1,0

– according to the values reported in the *Table I*: one initial placenta contains approximatively 4,8 grams of total lipids, that is to say: 3 grams of phospholipids and 0,9 gram of free fatty acids;
– according to the fatty acid composition of these two fractions reported in the last *Tables*, it represents about 500 mg of PUFAs (20:2 n-6 + 20:3 n-6 + 22:4 n-6 + 22:4 n-6 + 22:5 n-6 + 22:5 n-3 + 22:6 n-3) in phospholipids and 350 mg of PUFAs in free fatty acids.

This means that one placenta contains about 850 mg of PUFAs at the end of gestation.

If we do the same calculation for one placental tissue after blood elimination, we obtain 570 mg of PUFAs present in this fraction.

The main objective of the very preliminary study I will present now was to determine the fatty acid profile of red blood cell phospholipids of preterm infants at birth and to evaluate the influence of the gestational age. Three groups of infants were involved in the protocol. Eight infants born between 26 and 28 weeks of gestation, nine infants born between 30 and 32 weeks of gestation and eight term infants. Blood samples were obtained at birth before any blood transfusion, samples were collected in heparinized tubes to prevent coagulation and centrifuged to separate plasma and cells. After removal of plasma, erythrocytes were washed and lipids extracted according to a procedure of Folch.

The study of the fatty acid composition of red blood cell phospholipids from infants of various gestational age showed no significant difference of the two preterm infant groups (Table V). Relative levels of saturated fatty acids seem to be slightly higher in the term infant groups but statistical analyses are still in progress. This result suggests that the fatty acid status of the red cell membrane is not actually affected by the gestational age of the preterm infant at birth and that the polyunsaturated fatty acid content of red blood cell phospholipids in preterm infants will only decrease following birth if not adequate diet is administrated. Thank you for your attention.

Table V. Fatty acid composition of red blood cell phospholipids of infants at birth

Fatty acid	Preterm infants (n = 8) Gestational age = 26-28 weeks	Preterm infants (n = 9) Gestional age = 30-32 weeks	Term infants (n = 8)
C14:0	0,27 ± 0,24	0,32 ± 0,23	0,35 ± 0,04
DMA 16:0	2,21 ± 0,30	2,27 ± 0,32	2,62 ± 0,25
C16:0	20,07 ± 1,32	20,87 ± 1,70	23,21 ± 2,25
C16:1 N-9	0,65 ± 0,14	0,70 ± 0,18	0,53 ± 0,07
C16:1 N-7	1,11 ± 0,29	1,29 ± 0,68	0,65 ± 0,12
C17:0	0,45 ± 0,17	0,55 ± 0,18	0,57 ± 0,16
DMA 18:0	3,41 ± 0,40	3,01 ± 0,45	2,94 ± 0,26
C18:0	12,35 ± 1,22	11,45 ± 2,11	13,99 ± 0,73
C18:1 N-9	12,07 ± 1,04	11,01 ± 1,52	10,66 ± 0,90
C18:1 N-7	2,20 ± 0,26	2,16 ± 0,31	2,32 ± 0,21
C18:2 N-6	4,56 ± 0,70	5,35 ± 1,52	4,56 ± 0,56
C18:3 N-3	0,23 ± 0,23	0,33 ± 0,09	0,01 ± 0,02
C20:2 N-6	0,90 ± 0,20	1,13 ± 0,60	0,62 ± 0,24
C20:3 N-6	2,61 ± 0,36	2,75 ± 0,49	2,38 ± 0,53
C20:4 N-6	24,24 ± 1,51	23,50 ± 3,28	21,53 ± 2,05
C20:5 N-3	0,13 ± 0,15	0,11 ± 0,15	0,00 ± 0,00
C22:4 N-6	3,70 ± 0,46	3,48 ± 0,36	3,57 ± 0,68
C22:5 N-6	1,57 ± 0,18	1,50 ± 0,21	1,81 ± 0,41
C22:5 N-3	0,48 ± 0,05	0,80 ± 0,31	0,62 ± 0,13
C22:6 N-3	6,78 ± 0,66	7,42 ± 2,12	7,07 ± 1,13

Discussion

Chairman: Thank you very much for your presentation. The first question please.

J.M. Bourre: Just one comment and one question. This is human tissue. So according to this meeting, we are interested to have the formula with very long chain fatty acids. It means it will be to a certain extent cannibalism, because eating too many tissues. Are you aware of this problem or what about the psychological problem with the mother. Is there a different way to ingest human parts of human protein ? What about the cannibalism aspect of the situation? The question is, what about during extraction of occurrence of transisomers?

V. Chirouze: Yes, with the industrial process of blood extraction that didn't produce any sort of fatty acid isomers, we find exactly the same composition of fatty acid after and before blood extraction.

Chairman: In answer to this first question I'm sure he's aware that Merieux produces a whole series of materials which are injected into the children of Europe, so they're all cannibals in that sense. So the concept of human material going back into human materials is not novel.

C. Galli: You have reported a very detailed analysis of the fatty acids of erythrocytes at different stages, including very minor components. However apparently there is no eicosatrienoic acid in the n-9 series. Is that true that there is no n-9 in the erythrocytes?

V. Chirouze: In my analysis conditions I have not found this fatty acid.

Chairman: Could I ask technically of the placentas, what percentage of them is blood and what percentage is placental tissue? Of the blood, is it foetal blood or maternal blood in the vein?

V. Chirouze: After delivery I think in placenta there is always maternal blood and all this is frozen and then brought to the Merieux Institute where it is squeezed, still frozen, and then pressed. In residual tissue no blood remains.

Chairman: Yes, but in the blood that you extracted between the initial and the post, is it maternal blood you're taking out or is it mixture?

B. Salle : It's mainly maternal.

Chairman: It's mainly maternal blood, that's right but surely there is a little bit of blood coming from the foetus, but it's mainly the statement of what's in maternal blood. Any other comments or observations? Thank you very much indeed, Mrs Chirouze.

7

Fatty acids blood composition in foetal and maternal plasma

P. CRASTES de PAULET*, P. SARDA**, P. BOULOT***,
A. CRASTES de PAULET*

Laboratoire de Biochimie A*, Service de Néonatologie**
et Département d'Obstétrique***, CHU Lapeyronie, Montpellier, France

At birth, linoleic acid represents about 10% of the total fatty acids in cord plasma compared to 30% in maternal plasma, but surprisingly, arachidonate concentration in cord plasma is twice (($\simeq$10%)) that observed in the mother (($\simeq$5%). Similarly α-linolenate concentration in the newborn is half that in the mother (0.3% versus 0.6%), whereas C22:6 (n-3) concentration is double (3% versus 1.5%). This situation, specific to the newborn and never observed in adult, in which the relative plasma concentration of long chain polyunsaturated fatty acids (PUFA) exceeds that of their precursors, can be related to analogous observations on the fatty acid (FA) composition of plasma phospholipids made by Olegerd and Svennerholm [1] and de Lucchi *et al.* [2] on full term newborn infants and on the FA composition of the main lipid fractions by Friedman *et al.* [3, 4] in infants and in their mothers during the third trimester, at delivery.

It is obviously an extremely favourable situation for the development of the newborn, especially at a time when high quantities of C20:4 (n-6), and particularly of C22:6 (n-3), are needed by the brain and retina. However two questions arise: (1) What is (or are) the underlying mechanism(s) leading to this situation, at birth? (2) How does the situation envolve throughout gestation?

In this study we have attempted to answer this second question. To this end, we analyzed total lipid FA in plasma samples obtained from foetal cord and mothers between the 18th and 38th weeks of pregnancy. Plasma FA analysis was preferred to red blood cell FA analysis since FA distribution in plasma reflects the whole foetoplacental unit metabolism, expressed by lipoprotein synthesis and clearance, better than FA distribution in red blood cells, which, otherwise, is a better reflection of tissue composition in PUFA.

Subjects and methods

Subjects

For ethical and technical reasons, cord puncture on the umbilical vein was performed under strictly defined indications: (1) Detection of toxoplasm contamination of the foetus in cases of maternal seropositivity. (2) Foetal karyotyping in pregnant women over 38 years old in whom amniocentesis is no longer possible, or after echoscan detection of a malformation. (3) Foetal karyotyping when early hypotrophy is detected, in the absence of any evident etiology, particularly maternal hypertension.

Ninety six foetal blood samples were thus obtained, 71 of which were from absolutely normal foetuses. Simultaneously, 59 venous blood samples were obtained from the corresponding normal mothers.

For comparison, data obtained from 16 normal newborn babies (cord blood) and 17 non-pregnant women (mean age: 25 ± 4,5 years) are also reported. For the statistical analysis, observations were classified into four groups by increasing gestational age, as indicated in *Table I*.

Table I. Definition of experimental groups

Group	Gestational age (weeks)	Foetus (N)	Mothers (N)
1	18-22	23	15
2	23-27	21	18
3	28-32	16	14
4	33-37	12	12

Blood samples analysis

200 µl of blood, obtained from the umbilical vein by transabdominal puncture, under echoscan control, were collected in an heparinized microtube and immediately centrifuged at 3 000 g for 10 min. Plasma was kept frozen at – 20 °C until analysis. 1 ml of peripheral venous blood obtained from the mothers was similarly treated. Plasma lipids were extracted with chloroform/methanol 2:1 (v/v) by the Folch procedure [5]. FA were methylated by incubation for 30 min at 80 °C in methanol/sulfuric acid 19:1 (v/v). Fatty acid methyl esters were stored at – 20 °C under nitrogen until analysis by GLC using a Girdel 300 Delsi gas chromatograph equipped with a 25 m length × 0.32 mm fused silica capillary column FFAP*. Peaks were detected by FID and signals analysed using an ENICA 10 recorder/computer. Peaks were identified by comparison with known standards (Sigma). Results are reported as percent area.

---

* Nitroterephthalic ester of 20 M Carbowax (Chrompack-Middelburg NL).

Statistics

Differences between mean values to the different groups were assessed by a Student's t-test for compared data.

Results

Saturated fatty acids (SFA) (*Table II*)

Palmitic acid was, by far, the most abundant SFA in cord plasma at early gestation (group 1: 26.8%). Its level was significantly lower ($p < 10^{-5}$) than in newborn infants and rose progressively with gestational age. Throughout gestation, the same percentages were found in foetuses and in mothers. Interestingly, the levels in mothers were always significantly higher ($p < 10^{-2}$ to $< 10^{-5}$) than in non-pregnant women and increased in the third trimester: 31.2% in group 4 versus 25.1% in non-pregnant women.

Stearic acid: in foetuses, the level of stearic acid rose slowly with gestational age from 8.5% (group 1) to 9.6% (group 4), i.e. to the same percentage (9.8%) as in newborn infants. These levels (range 8.5% - 9.4%) were much higher than in mothers (6.4% - 5.5%). In mothers, the stearic acid level decreased significantly ($p < 10^{-3}$ to $< 10^{-5}$) during the last trimester (groups 3 and 4).

Lauric acid (data not shown): this is a "minor" SFA, both in foetuses and in mothers ($1.4 \pm 0.3\%$ and $1.6 \pm 0.3\%$ respectively) and we did not find any significant variation during gestation, neither in foetuses nor in mothers.

Mono unsaturated fatty acids (MUFA) (*Table II*)

Palmitoleic acid: as early as the end of the first trimester, and throughout gestation, significantly ($p < 10^{-5}$ to $< 10^{-2}$) higher levels of C16:1 (n-7) were observed in foetuses than in mothers (range 5.2%-6.5%, versus 2.9%-3.4%). These concentrations were in the same range in newborns. The levels in the third and fourth group of mothers were significantly higher ($p < 10^{-2}$) than in non-pregnant women.

Oleic acid: significantly much higher levels of C18:1 (n-9) were recorded in foetuses at the end of the 1st trimester, more than in mothers: 27.8% versus 19.8%. This level decreased with gestational age and, at the end of the gestation, was in the same range as in newborn infants and in non-pregnant women (22.1% versus respectively 20.7% and 18.8%). Mothers had the same levels of C18:1 (n-9) as non-pregnant women.

The marked elevation of MUFA and particularly C16:1 (n-7) in foetuses is characteristic of linoleic acid deficiency but, despite of careful examination of the chromatograms, and probably due to the high levels of C18:1 (n-9), we were unable to characterize any vaccenic acid, C18:1 (n-7), formed by elongation of C16:1 (n-7). However, its presence cannot be excluded.

Essential fatty acids and infant nutrition

Table II. Plasma total fatty acid distribution in foetuses (F) and mothers (M): main saturated and mono unsaturated fatty acids

FA		\multicolumn{6}{c}{Groups}					
		1	2	3	4	NB	NPW
C16:0	F	***** 26.8 ± 3.4	* 29.0 ± 3.3	30.5 ± 2.9	30.7 ± 2.6	31.8 ± 3.2	
	M	•• 27.4 ± 2.0	••• 28.2 ± 1.9	•••• 29.2 ± 2.6	••••• 31.2 ± 3.1		25.1 ± 2.6
C18:0	F	* 8.5 ± 1.7 ↑ 10^{-3} ↓	** 8.6 ± 0.8 ↑ $< 10^{-5}$ ↓	8.8 ± 1.8 ↑ $< 10^{-5}$ ↓	9.6 ± 1.0 ↑ $< 10^{-5}$ ↓	9.8 ± 1.3	
	M	6.4 ± 1.9	6.2 ± 1.7	••••• 5.2 ± 0.7	••• 5.5 ± 0.8		7.3 ± 1.6
C16:1 (n-7)	F	5.3 ± 2.0 ↑ 10^{-4} ↓	5.2 ± 2 ↑ 10^{-4} ↓	* 6.5 ± 2.4 ↑ $< 10^{-5}$ ↓	5.6 ± 2.1 ↑ 10^{-2} ↓	4.8 ± 1.1	
	M	3.1 ± 1.0	2.9 ± 1.0	•• 3.1 ± 0.6	•• 3.4 ± 1.1		2.5 ± 0.7
C18:1 (n-9)	F	***** 27.8 ± 4.3 ↑ $< 10^{-5}$ ↓	**** 25.5 ± 4 ↑ $< 10^{-5}$ ↓	** 23.2 ± 2.6 ↑ $< 10^{-5}$ ↓	22.1 ± 1.8	20.7 ± 2.3	
	M	19.8 ± 1.7	19.2 ± 2.3	20.8 ± 2.7	20.9 ± 2.8		18.8 ± 3.3

Statistically different from newborn infants (NB) at $p < 10^{-5}$ (*****), $p < 10^{-4}$ (****), $p < 10^{-3}$ (***), $p < 10^{-2}$ (**), $p < 0.05$ (*).
Statistically different from non-pregnant women (NPW) at $p < 10^{-5}$ (•••••), $p < 10^{-4}$ (••••), $p < 10^{-3}$ (•••), $p < 10^{-2}$ (••), $p < 0.05$ (•).
↑ $< 10^{-5}$ ↓, ↑ 10^{-4} ↓, ↑ 10^{-3} ↓: statistically different between foetuses and mothers of the same group.

Polyunsaturated fatty acids (PUFA)

A) (n-6) series (*Table IIIA*)

Linoleic acid: the very low levels of C18:2 (n-6), already observed in newborn infants, were apparent in foetuses as early as the end of the first trimester (9.0% versus 29.6% in mothers of the same group). Large individual variations were noted both in the foetuses and in the mothers but, interestingly, foetus and mother values

Table IIIA. Plasma total fatty acid distribution in foetuses (F) and mothers (M): main (n-6) polyunsaturated fatty acids

FA		Groups					
		1	2	3	4	NB	NPW
C18:2 (n-6)	F	**** 9.0 ± 2.1 ↑ 10^{-3} ↓	* 10.1 ± 2.9 ↑ 10^{-3} ↓	** 9.8 ± 1.7 ↑ 10^{-3} ↓	10.7 ± 2.6 ↑ 10^{-3} ↓	12.1 ± 2.2	
	M	29.6 ± 4.1	27.4 ± 3.5	•• 28.1 ± 3.3	•• 26.4 ± 4.5		31.3 ± 5.1
C20:3 (n-6)	F	***** 1.1 ± 0.5	***** 1.2 ± 0.6	** 1.7 ± 0.5	** 1.4 ± 0.8	2.5 ± 1.0	
	M	1.0 ± 0.5	• 1.3 ± 0.5	NS 1.3 ± 0.6	• 1.3 ± 0.5		0.9 ± 0.4
C20:4 (n-6)	F	10.1 ± 2.6 ↑ $< 10^{-5}$ ↓	11.5 ± 2.7 ↑ $< 10^{-5}$ ↓	11.5 ± 3 ↑ $< 10^{-5}$ ↓	11.1 ± 2.4 ↑ $< 10^{-5}$ ↓	11.2 ± 2.7	
	M	5.0 ± 1.4	5.7 ± 1.4	5.1 ± 1.0	•• 4.4 ± 0.8		5.5 ± 1.3

were correlated (*figure 1*): throughout gestation, the percentage of C18:2 (n-6) in total plasma lipids in the foetus was a third of the concentration in the mother. In mothers, the concentrations were in the same range or slightly below those in the non-pregnant women.

γ-linolenic acid (data not shown): the levels were very low, both in foetuses and mothers, and in the same range (0.2%) as in newborn infants or in non-pregnant women.

Dihomo-γ-linolenic acid: concentrations in foetuses were in the same range as in mothers or in non-pregnant women (1.1% to 1.7% versus 1.0% to 1.3%), but significantly lower than in newborn infants (2.5%).

Arachidonic acid: the very high levels of C20:4 (n-6), characteristic of newborn infants, were observed in foetuses as early as the end of the first trimester. They remained constant ($\simeq$ 10% of total FA) during gestation, and can be compared to the $\simeq$ 5% concentration observed in mothers, which is in the same range as that measured in non-pregnant women.

B) (n-3) series (*Table IIIB*)

α-linolenic acid (data not shown): the percentage was lower in foetuses ($\cong$ 0.3%) (similar values as recorded in newborn infants) than in mothers (($\simeq$ 0.6%), with no significant variations during gestation.

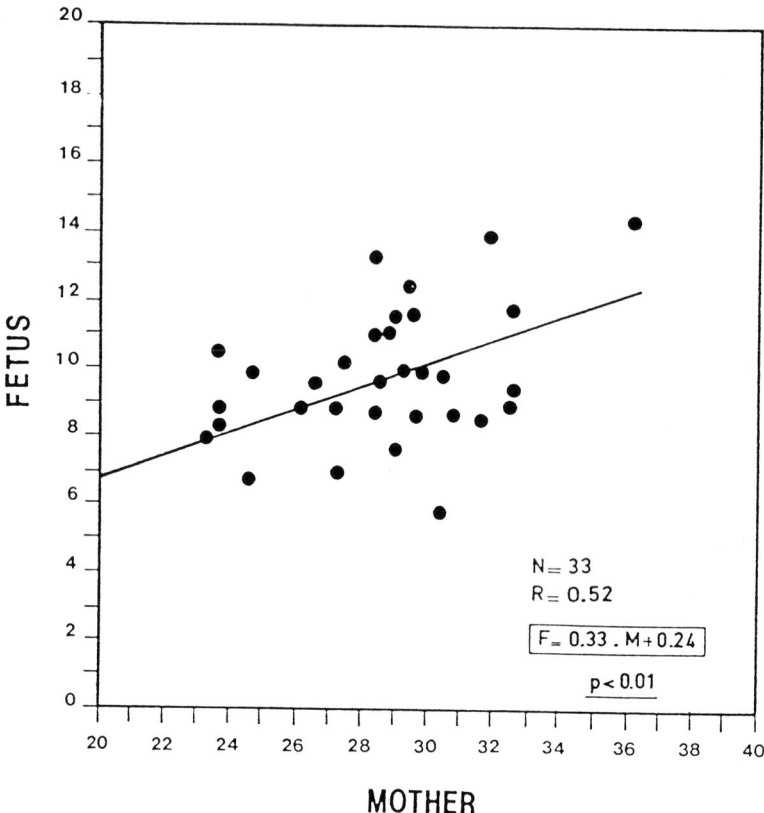

Figure 1. Total lipid fatty acids 18:2 (n–6).

Eicosapentaenoic acid (EPA): the percentages of C20:5 (n-3) were low, with no difference between foetuses and mothers. They were clearly higher in foetuses of the first group than in newborn infants (0.5% versus 0.1%). In mothers, they were lower in groups 3 and 4 than in non-pregant women (0.1% versus 0.4%).

Docosahexaenoic acid (DHA): C22:6 (n-3) was by far the main PUFA of the n-3 series both in foetuses and mothers. As for C20:4 (n-6), the high levels observed in newborn infants (2.5%) were recorded as early as the end of the first trimester (2.4%) with small decrease in groups 3 and 4. Until the 28th week, levels were significantly higher in foetuses than in mothers (2.4% – 2.0% versus 1.5% – 1.4%) in whom levels were in the same range as in non-pregnant women. The concentration of DHA remained higher in the foetuses of groups 3 and 4, compared with mothers, but with no significant difference, due to large individual variations.

Table IIIB. Plasma total fatty acid distribution in foetuses (F) and mothers (M): main (n-3) polyunsaturated fatty acids

FA		\multicolumn{6}{c}{Groups}					
		1	2	3	4	NB	NPW
C20:5 (n-3)	F	* 0.5 ± 0.8	0.1 ± 0.2	0.1 ± 0.1	0.1 ± 0.2	0.1 ± 0.1	
	M	• 0.3 ± 0.3	••• 0.2 ± 0.2	••••• 0.1 ± 0.1	•• 0.1 ± 0.1		0.4 ± 0.2
C22:6 (n-3)	F	2.4 ± 1.1 ↑ < 10^{-5} ↓	2.0 ± 0.9 ↑ < 10^{-5} ↓	* (5%) 1.9 ± 0.6	** 1.8 ± 0.5	2.5 ± 0.6	
	M	1.5 ± 0.9	1.3 ± 0.6	1.5 ± 0.5	1.5 ± 0.6		1.6 ± 0.7

For Tables IIIA and IIIB the same symbols as in Table II are used.

Discussion

The main conclusions that can be drawn from this study are the following:
- The characteristic biological pattern observed in newborn infants, i.e., low levels of essential "precursor" fatty acids (PFA), C18:2 (n-6) and C18:3 (n-3), and high levels of "daughter" fatty acids (DFA), mainly C20:4 (n-6) and C22:6 (n-3) respectively, was also manifest in foetuses as early as the end of the first trimester of gestation.
- The very low levels of C18:2 (n-6) stand in contrast to the almost "normal" values observed in the mothers, relative to non-prenant women. Nevertheless, there is a good correlation between the values in foetuses (F) and mothers (M), F = 0.33 (M) + 0.24 ($p < 0.01$).
- These very low levels of C18:2 (n-6) could explain the high concentrations of MUFA, particularly C16:1 (n-7), observed in the foetuses mainly at the end of the first trimester but also throughout gestation: linoleic acid is known to inhibit Δ9-desaturase. However, in spite of this apparent "biologically" severe esential fatty acid (EFA) deficiency, neither high levels of Mead acid (C20:3 (n-9)) nor low levels of arachidonic acid were observed. On the contrary, arachidonic acid reached an unexpectedly high concentration which was twice that in the mother!

Our observations on the contribution of Mead acid to total plasma lipids differ from the data by Friedman [4] who recorded high levels of C20:3 (n-9) (up to 2.5% at the end of gestation) in plasma phospholipids. Higher levels of Mead acid would perhaps be found in foetal arterial rather than in venous plasma, in which the FA composition is modified by placental activities. Indeed, at delivery the EFA status of human umbilical arteries is poorer than that of umbilical veins, as recently shown by Hornstra et al. [6].

- The high leels of DFA, C22:6 (n-3) and mainly C20:4 (n-6), observed early in gestation and during growth of the normal foetuses are noteworthy. Our earlier data on hypotrophic foetuses clearly showed that these high levels of C20:4 (n-6) and C22:6 (n-3) provide a very good indication of normal foetal development [7].

The above data thus clearly show that the biological pattern of distribution of PUFA which characterizes newborn plasma lipids is observed very early in gestation. High levels of C20:4 (n-6) and C22:6 (n-3) correlate with normal growth of the foetus. These data, however, beg the question: what could be the mechanism(s) for such high levels of DFA in spite of very low levels of parent PUFA. Obviously the EFA C18:2 (n-6) and C18:3 (n-3) are supplied by the mother, but two main mechanisms could explain the high DFA levels in foetal blood: (1) selective transfer or secretion by the placenta of maternal DFA; (2) high activity of the desaturases and elongase in foeto-placental unit.

Selective transfer or secretion

The human placenta, like other hemochorial placentas, is permeable to free fatty acid (FFA). The supply of maternal blood FFA to the human foetus has been extensively studied, and recently "revisited" by Hull et al. [8,9], either through perfusion of placental lobes with [^{14}C] FA or analysis of umbilical vein-artery differences in FFA after elective caesarean section. According to Hull [9], with the exception of oleic acid and arachidonic acid, the transfer of FFA across the maternal plasma is non-selective, depending on the concentration in the maternal plasma. Although the umbilical vein-artery difference obtained for DHA would be largely sufficient to cover the requirements for brain growth, the situation for free arachidonic acid is quite different, the arterio-venous gradient being small and negatively correlated to maternal venous plasma level.

However, it is clear that the high levels of total C22:6 (n-3) or C20:4 (n-6) cannot simply be explained by high levels or their free form. A selective placental secretion, mainly in phospholipids, of these DFA picked up from maternal FFA, triglycerides, or phospholipids, must be taken into account. Using the placental lobe perfusion technique, Kuhn and Crawford [10] have shown that free [^{14}C]-arachidonic acid, when injected into the maternal arterial circulation, is preferentially incorporated into phosphoglycerides for export into the foetal circulation. The non-transfer to the foetus of [^{14}C]-arachidonic acid when in 2-position of lecithin, as observed by these authors, is surprising, since high phospholipase A_2 activity is observed in human placenta: this high activity could be involved in PG biosynthesis and secretion directed to the maternal circulation, as suggested by Kuhn and Crawford [10].

Interestingly, high lipoprotein lipase activity has also been found in placenta [11]. This enzyme could also be involved in the transfer of maternal FA, for instance, in the metabolism of maternal VLDL triglycerides, or artificial emulsions.

All of these results are consistent with the observations of Coleman [12] on the activities of enzymes involved in triacylglycerol and phosphatidylcholine biosynthesis in the rat placenta, but data on placental enzymes and maternal PUFA secretion in foetal phospholipids or triglycerides under physiological conditions are sadly lacking in humans.

Fatty acids blood composition in foetal and maternal plasma

Desaturases and elongase activities in the foeto-placental unit

According to Chambaz *et al.* [13], human placenta has no detectable Δ5- and Δ6-desaturase activities. This result is in agreement with the observation of Booth [8] that [^{14}C]-γ-linolenic acid is not converted into [^{14}C] arachidonic acid by perfused lobes of human placenta. On the other hand, they found high Δ5- and Δ6- activities in the liver of one 18 week and two 22 week foetuses [13], which were closed to those reported by others in adult liver [14]. Despite this result and because of the low arachidonate concentration in foetal liver microsomes, compared to plasma, they concluded that arachidonic acid is supplied to the foetus through a preferential transfer across the placenta. We do not entirely share this view since the relative mass of 3rd trimester foetal liver is such that it could be involved in DFA metabolism. Moreover indirect pathophysiological evidence is given for our contention by the slow decrease in DFA in plasma phospholipids after delivery [15] in newborn infants fed with milk formula containing normal EFA but very low C20:4 (n-6) and C22:6 (n-3) and by the low DFA levels in hypotrophic newborn infants from mothers with no maternal hypertension [7].

The situation could be over simplified as shown in *figure 2*. The exclusive role of placental transfer and selective secretion of DFA, operative at the beginning of gestation, could progressively be taken over by foetal metabolism. But since foetal liver desaturases-elongase chain reaction has not been clearly demonstrated in physiological conditions, this remains hypothetical.

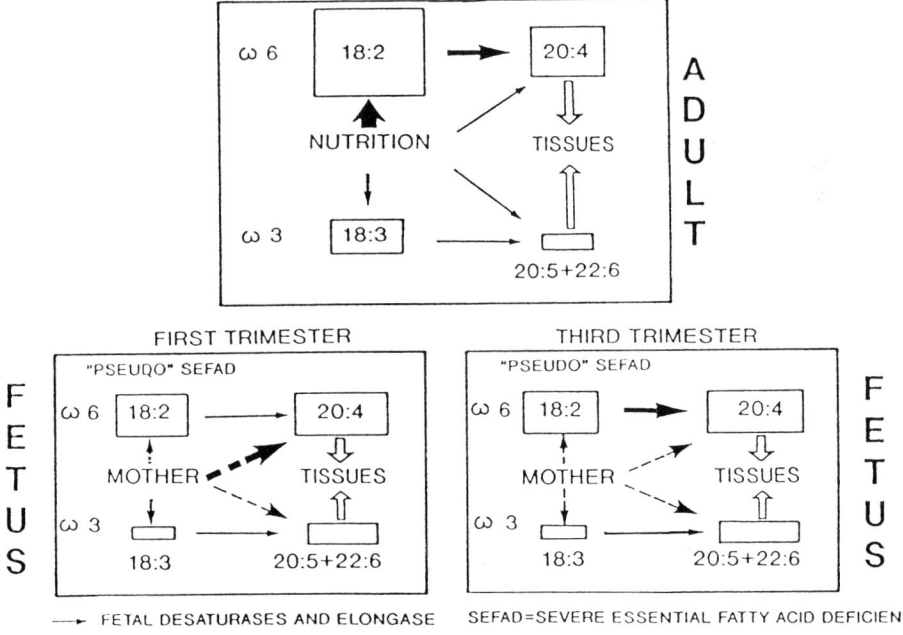

Figure 2. EFAs and long chain EFAs in adult and foetus.

We are currently trying to determine this pathway and its importance in normal and premature newborn infants, using deuterated PUFA and an analytical methodology similar to the one we have previously used in adults [16].

Acknowledgments

Benjamin Limasset is gratefully acknowledged for his valuable assistance in the statistical analysis.

References

1. Olegerd R., Svennerholm L. (1970) Fatty acid composition of plasma and red cell phosphoglycerides in full term infant and their mothers. *Acta Paediatr Scand* 59:637-47.
2. de Lucchi C., Pita M.L., Fauss M.J., Periago J.L., Gil A. (1987) Changes in the fatty acid composition of plasma and red blood cell membrane during the first hours of life in human neonates. *Early Hum Dev* 15:85-93.
3. Friedman Z., Danon A., Lamberth E.L., Mann W.J. (1978) Cord blood fatty acid composition in infants and in their mothers during the third trimester. *J Pediatr* 92:461-6.
4. Friedman Z. (1987) Essential fatty acid requirements for term and preterm infants. In: Horisberger M., Bracco U., eds. Nestlé Nutrition Workshop Series, vol. 13, Nestlé Nutrition. New York: Raven Press, 79-92.
5. Folch J., Lees M., Sloane Stanley G.H. (1957) A simple method for the isolation and purification of total lipids from animal tissues. *J Biol Chem* 226:497-509.
6. Hornstra G., Van Houwelingen A.C., Simonis M., Gerrard J.M. (1989) Fatty acid composition of umbilical arteries and veins: possible implications for the fetal EFA-status. *Lipids* 24:511-7.
7. Sarda P., Boulot P., Crastes de Paulet P., Rieu D., Bonnet H., Crastes de Paulet A. (1989) Acides gras des lipides totaux chez le fœtus hypotrophique après la 20e semaine de gestation. 19e Congrès International de Pédiatrie, Paris, 23-28/7/89, Abstr. 0-19, 417.
8. Booth C., Elphick M.C., Hendrickse W., Hull D. (1981) Investigation of [^{14}C] linoleic acid conversion into [^{14}C] arachidonic acid and placental transfer of linoleic acid and palmiti acids across the perfused human placenta. *J Dev Physiol* 3:177-89.
9. Hendrickse W., Stammers J.P., Hull D. (1985) The transfer of free fatty acids across the human placenta. *Br J Obstet Gynaecol* 92:945-52.
10. Kuhn D.C., Crawford M. (1986) Placental essential fatty acid transport and prostaglandin synthesis. *Prog Lipid Res* 25:345-53.
11. Biale Y. (1985) Lipolytic activity in the placentas of chronically deprived fetuses. *Acta Obstet Gynecol Scand* 64:111-4.
12. Coleman R.A. (1986) Placental metabolism and transport of lipid. *Fed Proc* 45 (10):2519-23.
13. Chambaz J., Ravel D., Manier M.C., Pepin D., Mulliez N., Béréziat G. (1985) Essential fatty acids interconversion in the human fetal liver. *Biol Neonate* 47:136-40.
14. De Gomez Dumm I.N.T., Brenner R.R. (1975) Oxidative desaturation of γ-linolenic and stearic acids by human liver microsomes. *Lipids* 10:315-7.

15. Gil A., Lozano E., de Lucchi C., Maldonado J., Molina J.A., Pita M. (1988) Changes in the fatty acid profiles of plasma lipid fractions induced by dietary nucleotides in infants born at term. *Eur J Clin Nutr* 42:473-81.
16. El Boustani S., Causse J.E., Descomps B., Monnier L., Mendy F., Crastes de Paulet A. (1989) Direct *in vivo* characterisation of delta 5 desaturase activity in humans by deuterium labelling: effect of insulin. *Metabolism* 38: 315-21.

Discussion

Chairman: Thank you very much indeed. Questions and observations, please.

B. Koletzko: Congratulations for this very elegant study. I think that this other fact has been shown and placenta selectively utilized lipid fractions from maternal blood.

A. Crastes de Paulet: And so, you think there is no direct transfer of linoleic acid from placenta? It is only for arachidonic acid, not linoleic acid. This is your opinion, or has that been demonstrated clearly?

B. Koletzko: There is some data available showing that there would be a selective maternal foetal transfer of long chain polyunsaturated fatty acids.

A. Crastes de Paulet: Yes, but if this phenomenon is important, immediately after delivery there should be a dramatic decrease in the concentration of arachidonic acid and docosahexaenoic acid. Yet we never find this decrease.

Chairman: May I just express an anxiety I have about the discussion? The free fatty acids come from different compartments, and the compartment concerned with transfer is the free fatty acid compartment. You measured fatty acid distribution in the total lipid fractions which will include the free fatty acid and fatty acids from the endogenous triglycerides.
The relative proportions of free fatty acids and of the endogenous triglyceride fatty acids are going to be very different in the maternal circulation and in the newborn. So really one wants to know the breakdown of these compartments, because the one that's really vital for placental transfer is the free fatty acids and we've shown quite clearly that there is a correlation between maternal and foetal linoleic acid at term at least.

A. Crastes de Paulet: Yes, I agree with your comment, but we analysed whole lipids FA distribution because it is very difficult to analyse the different lipid classes, due to the very small sample.

Chairman: I think you did marvelously to study it at all because you have the handicap of not being able to break it down into the various fatty acids.

A. Crastes de Paulet: It is impossible to analyse the free fatty acids with so small amount of blood.

Chairman: But that would distort it a lot because the relative distribution of fatty acids into those different compartments is different.

B. Koletzko: May I just make a comment on that point. I think it has to be more emphasized because it has been shown that free fatty acids in the foetus are immediately incorporated selectively in foetal phospholipids and if we looked at just concentrations of free fatty acids in the maternal and foetal blood, we certainly cannot understand correctly the phenomena of transfer that occur.

S. Carlson: Yes, I guess I would like to express the same concern as Dr Koletzko's. I think once the babies are separated from mother, we clearly see a defined drop of arachidonic acid and docosahexanoic acid unless they are incorporated into the diet.

J.M. Bourre: What about the distribution of the lipoproteins in the foetus in human or in other species? It could be possible that in fact an increased amount of the long chain fatty acids could be due either to changes of the proportion between the lipoproteins or could be due to increase the amount of phospholipids in these lipoproteins. In this case I would like to come back to what we are speaking about which is the free fatty acids. It is not sure that all fatty acids which are transported or taken are those which are free. It could be possible that those which are used are coming from the phospholipids. These could mean that in fact those fatty acids in the phospholipids are the one which are found afterwards in all the membranes, including the brain for instance.

A. Crastes de Paulet: So if I understand your question, we have to separate lipoproteins from cord blood and analyse separately their FA? But you have to realize that there it is a big problem to obtain sufficient samples: 200 microlitres of whole blood is a maximum we can obtain.

J.M. Bourre: But, I know, maybe just in comparison to other species. I don't know, otherwise we have to choose live monkeys.

A. Crastes de Paulet: I would like to say that it is a preliminary study and we have been very strongly surprised by the results we have obtained. I think that anyway there is a crucial question we would like to be answered: why did we never find the Mead acid in cord blood total lipids, in spite of a very low level of linoleic acid and of a very high level of $\Delta 9$-desaturase activity, as strongly suspected by the high levels of palmitoleic acid? Dealing with essential fatty acid metabolism, the situation of the foetus looks like an essential fatty acid deficiency, but with an incomprehensible absence of Mead's acid! Why? I put the question on the table!

8

Human milk and fatty acids: quantitative aspects

G. KOHN

*Milupa AG, Bahnstrasse,
D-6382 Friedrichsdorf/Ts, Germany*

In human milk the lipid fraction accounts for about 60% of the energy for the young infant. But besides this energetic aspects some constituents of human milk lipids like the essential fatty acids with a chain length of C18 and the very long-chain polyunsaturated fatty acids with 20 and 22 carbon atoms (VLC-PUFA) might be of special physiological importance in early human life.

In the following it will be focused on the latter type of the very long-chain polyunsaturated fatty acids, named VLC-PUFA's, that means that it deals with the group of the ω6-desaturated VLC-PUFA's, with eicosatrienoic and arachidonic acid as main components and the ω3-desaturated VLC-PUFA's with eicosapentaenoic and docosahexaenoic acid. The VLC-PUFA's of the ω6- and ω3-family are derived from the essential fatty acids linoleic and alpha-linolenic acid by further carboxyl-directed desaturation and elongation. However, there is still a discussion about the activity of the desaturating and elongating enzymes in term and preterm human infants (Clandinin *et al.*, 1980; Chambaz *et al.*, 1985, Koletzko, 1986; Pita *et al.*, 1988).

VLC-PUFA's have essential biological functions as precursors of eicosanoids (van Dorp, 1964; Koletzko, 1986; Seyberth and Kühl, 1988). On the other hand, VLC-PUFA's - due to their structural role as part of the phospholipids - affect the fluidity and stability of biomembranes and the activity of membrane bound enzymes (Crawford *et al.*, 1981; Koletzko, 1986). Especially the biomembranes of the neural tissues of brain and retina are rich in both ω6- and ω3-VLC-PUFA's. The high need of phospholipids and VLC-PUFA's during the last trimester of pregnancy and during postnatal myelinization may suggest their importance for the term and preterm newborn infant. These aspects of the physiological importance of VLC-PUFA's and their placental transfer have been discussed elsewhere before.

The requirement of the young infant for VLC-PUFA's is met by appreciable amounts (1,7 wt%) of these fatty acids in human milk (*Table I*). The results shown represent mean values for mature human milk in Germany and were published by Koletzko *et al.*, (1988). In contrast to human milk cow's milk, as a widely used basis for infant formulas, contains only very small amounts of arachidonic and eicosapentaenoic acid. Also goat milk is poor in these fatty acids. The milk from platypus might be a source for VLC-PUFA, due to their relatively high content of VLC-PUFA's, but unfortunately there are only small volumes available of the milk of this egg-laying animal from Australia.

Table I. The fatty acid composition [wt%] of human, cow, goat and platypus milk

Fatty Acids	Milk			
	Human[1]	Cow[2]	Goat[3]	Platypus[4]
C12-0	4.4	5.2	2.3	ND
C14-0	6.7	14.0	8.7	1.6
C16-0	21.8	31.0	26.5	19.8
C18-0	8.1	8.1	10.3	3.9
C18-1ω9	34.3	17.8	25.0	22.7
C18-2ω6	10.8	1.6	2.6	5.4
C18-3ω3	0.8	1.4	1.7	7.6
C20-2ω6	0.34	ND	0.10	0.50
C20-3ω6	0.26	ND	ND	0.20
C20-4ω6	0.36	0.11	0.34	2.40
C22-2ω6	0.11	ND	ND	ND
C22-4ω6	0.08	ND	ND	0.40
C22-5ω6	ND	ND	ND	ND
C20-5ω3	0.04	0.08	0.05	4.50
C22-5ω3	0.17	0.12	ND	4.20
C22-6ω3	0.22	ND	tr	tr

Abbr.: ND = not detected; tr = traces.
[1] adapted from Koletzko *et al.* (1988)
[2] adapted from Hagemeister *et al.* (1988)
[3] adapted from Sawaya *et al.* (1984)
[4] adapted from Gibson *et al.* (1988)

In recent reviews on human milk lipids (Jensen *et al.*, 1978; Jensen *et al.*, 1980; Ferris and Jensen, 1984; Picciano, 1984) several authors discussed the lack of reliable data on the content and composition of human milk lipids due to improper sampling techniques, different methods of sample storage and different methods for the extraction and determination of lipids and fatty acids. In several studies also in our company it could be shown that inter- and intra-individual differences in the lipid content and fatty acid composition of human milk occur depending on diurnal changes, feeding phase (for/hindmilk), age of lactation, left or right breast and the nutritional status of the mother. Although in recent years much analytical work has been done on human milk, there is still a special need for consistant and detailed data of the content of VLC-PUFA's in human milk. It should be pointed out that questions on the concentrations of minor components like the VLC-PUFA's and also the eicosanoids in human milk need detailed information on the method of sample collection, the nutritional background of the mother and the analyzing procedures.

In the following, results are reviewed, which were published by the research division of our company (Harzer et al., 1984, 1986): on the content of VLC-PUFA's in term human milk during lactation, their content in different lipid classes and in comparison between term and preterm human milk. In these studies the different samples of human milk were taken at all nursing times throughout the sampling day by complete emptying of both breasts into sterile containers using an electric breast pump. Each milk sample was mixed and a portion of about 20 ml was removed, immediately deep frozen and stored below minus 30 degrees centigrade. The total lipids were extracted by a modified Folch-method and the fatty acid pattern was determined by capillary gas chromatography.

To study the changes in the lipid content and fatty acid pattern during the early phases of lactation 550 milk samples from healthy mothers of term infants were analyzed at seven times between the first and 36th day of lactation.

The triglycerides of the term human milk, that account for 96 to 99% of the total lipids, increased from 1.9 to about 3.5 grams per 100 ml mainly during the first week postpartum and remained more or less constant thereafter (*figure 1*). There are appreciable interindividual variations in the triglyceride content of the different sampling days. In contrast, the cholesterol concentration decreased from 35 to 20 mg/100 ml, whereas the phospholipids remained more or less constant at 40 mg/100 ml all throughout lactation.

On the basis of the total lipid content and the relative amount of each fatty acid (weight % of total fatty acids) the absolute amounts of VLC-PUFA's were calculated. The first line of *Table II* repeats the development of the total lipid content from 1.9 (at the beginning) to 3.9 g/100 ml at the end of the analyzed period. During this phase of lactation there is a marked decrease in the relative content of the total VLC-PUFA's from 3.7 wt% at the beginning of colostrum to 1.5 wt% in mature term human milk. In relation to the total lipid content the absolute content of VLC-PUFA's amounts to 46.3 to 72.2 mg/100 ml. Due to the increase in the total lipid content and due to the interindividual standard deviations there is only a small decrease in the absolute amount of VLC-PUFA's during lactation. The results indicate that there is slightly larger decrease in the content of ω3-VLC-PUFA's during lactation, so that the ratio of ω6- to ω3-VLC-PUFA's increases from 2.4 to 4.6. A similar decrease in the relative content of VLC-PUFA's in term human milk during lactation has been published by Bitman et al. (1983).

Separating the total lipids from term human milk into the triglyceride and phospholipid fraction shows that the relative content of VLC-PUFA's is much higher in the polar lipids (*Table III*).

The phospholipids contain 11.3 wt% of VLC-PUFA's and the triglycerides only 1.5 wt%. Especially the concentrations of arachidonic and docosahexaenoic acid are more than ten times higher in the phospholipid than in the triglyceride fraction. But

Essential fatty acids and infant nutrition

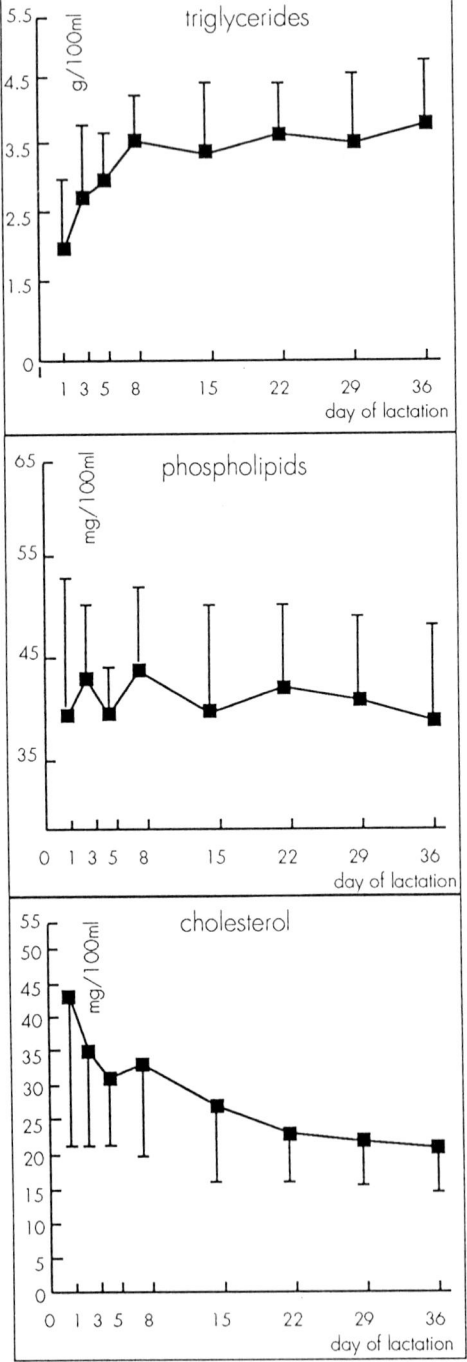

Figure 1. Changing patterns of human milk lipids during lactation; means ± SD (adapted from Harzer *et al.*, 1983).

Table II. The content of total lipids and VLC-PUFA's in term human milk during lactation

	Day of lactation							
	1	3	5	8	15	22	29	36
Total Lipids [g/100 ml]	1.9 ± 0.8	2.8 ± 0.8	2.9 ± 0.6	3.6 ± 0.6	3.5 ± 0.8	3.7 ± 0.6	3.6 ± 0.9	3.9 ± 1
cal. VLC-PUFA (rel.) [wt%]	3.70	2.67	2.36	2.14	1.63	1.33	1.63	1.46
cal. VLC-PUFA (abs.) [mg/100 ml]	67.6	70.3	64.4	72.2	53.8	46.3	55.9	53.7
cal. ω6-VLC-PUFA (abs.) [mg/100ml]	47.9	50.6	48.9	53.3	41.2	36.3	44.0	44.2
cal. ω3-VLC-PUFA (abs.) [mg/100ml]	19.8	19.8	15.5	19.0	12.6	10.0	11.8	9.5
$R = \dfrac{\omega 6\text{-VLC-PUFA}}{\omega 3\text{-VLC-PUFA}}$	2.42	2.52	3.16	2.81	3.28	3.62	3.71	4.65

Abbr.: cal. = calculated; rel. = relative; abs. = absolute; R = ratio

since 96 to 99% of the total lipids from term human milk are triglycerides, about 90% of the VLC-PUFA's available for the breastfed infant derive from the neutral lipid fraction. The work of Hundreiser et al. (1983) indicates that the phospholipids PE and PC contain VLC-PUFA's predominately at position C2 of the glycerol backbone. Although Weber et al. (1988) recently could separate the total triglyceride fraction of human milk into 94 molecular species, no results are available for the minor fatty acid fraction of VLC-PUFA's according to their positional distribution at the triglyceride molecule or the type of VLC-PUFA-triglycerides.

The separation of phospholipids into phospholipid subclasses by Bitman et al. (1984) and also in our laboratory (Haug et al., 1983) indicates that especially PE, PS and PI are rich in VLC-PUFA's, whereas sphingomyelin contains only small amounts or is probably free of these fatty acids.

As mentioned before the supply with very long-chain polyunsaturated fatty acids might be of special benefit for the premature human infant (Clandinin et al., 1980; Crawford et al.,1981; Koletzko, 1986). A comparison of preterm and term human milk during three phases of lactation is given in *Table IV*. Results for colostrum, transitional and mature human milk were calculated on the basis of daily mean values of 14 mothers who delivered before the 35th week of gstation.

In addition to the results from term human milk with a decrease in the relative content of total VLC-PUFA's from 2.9 to 1.5 wt%, also in preterm human milk the VLC-PUFA's are higher in colostrum and lower in transitional and mature milk. It

Table III. The content of VLC-PUFA's in the triglyceride and phospholipid fraction of term human milk (36th day of lactation)*

Fatty acid	Triglycerides	Phospholipids
C20-2ω6	0.35	0.39
C20-3ω6	0.30	1.95
C20-4ω6	0.39	5.77
C22-2ω6	0.12	0.19
C22-4ω6	0.05	0.34
C22-5ω6	tr	0.10
ω6-VLC-PUFA's	1.21	8.74
C20-5ω3	0.05	0.25
C22-5ω3	0.05	0.35
C22-6ω3	0.16	2.00
ω3-VLC-PUFA's	0.26	2.60
ω6-VLC-PUFA's + ω3-VLC-PUFA's	1.47	11.34

* adapted from Harzer and Haug (1984); Daily means (wt%); n = 17; tr = traces

Table IV. The concentrations [wt%] of VLC-PUFA's in term and preterm human milk during lactation (C = colostrum, T = transitional, M = mature)*

	C 1-6d	T 7-18d	M 19-36d	
calc. VLC-PUFA (rel.)	2.91	1.89	1.47	term
	3.58	2.31	2.66	preterm
calc. ω6-VLC-PUFA (rel.)	2.11	1.41	1.18	term
	2.98	1.84	2.19	preterm
calc. ω3-VLC-PUFA (rel.)	0.80	0.47	0.30	term
	0.61	0.47	0.47	preterm

* calculated from Harzer (1986) and Harzer et al. (1983)

should be pointed out that the concentration of VLC-PUFA's is higher in preterm than in term human milk. This is especially the case in the content of ω6-VLC-PUFA's whereas the ω3-VLC-PUFA's do not show remarkable differences between term and preterm human milk.

The results published by Bitman *et al.* (1983) demonstrate a higher content both in ω6- *and* ω3-VLC-PUFA's in very preterm human milk (VPT) and preterm human milk (PT) compared to term human milk (T) (*figure 2*). Especially the colostrum shows marked differences between very preterm and preterm milk and term milk on the other hand. All the three gestational groups show reduced concentrations of VLC-PUFA's with increasing lactational age. The authors conclude from these observations that "the elevated levels of long chain polyunsaturated fatty acids in preterm milk may be of special benefit for the needs of premature infants".

Finally some literature results on the content of eicosanoids and primarily on the content of prostaglandins in human milk should be discussed. Several authors especially studied prostaglandins in human milk, because of the possible beneficial effect of prostaglandins on the gastro-intestinal tract of the human infant (Friedman, 1986).

Prostaglandins, thromboxanes and leukotrienes are derived from VLC-PUFA's. The reaction pathway for the biosynthesis of eicosanoids starts with the liberation of VLC-PUFA's from a phospholipid molecule of the membrane bilayer by the action of a phospholipase. The free VLC-PUFA's can be metabolized to the group of leukotrienes by the action of a lipoxygenase or by the action of a cyclooxygenase

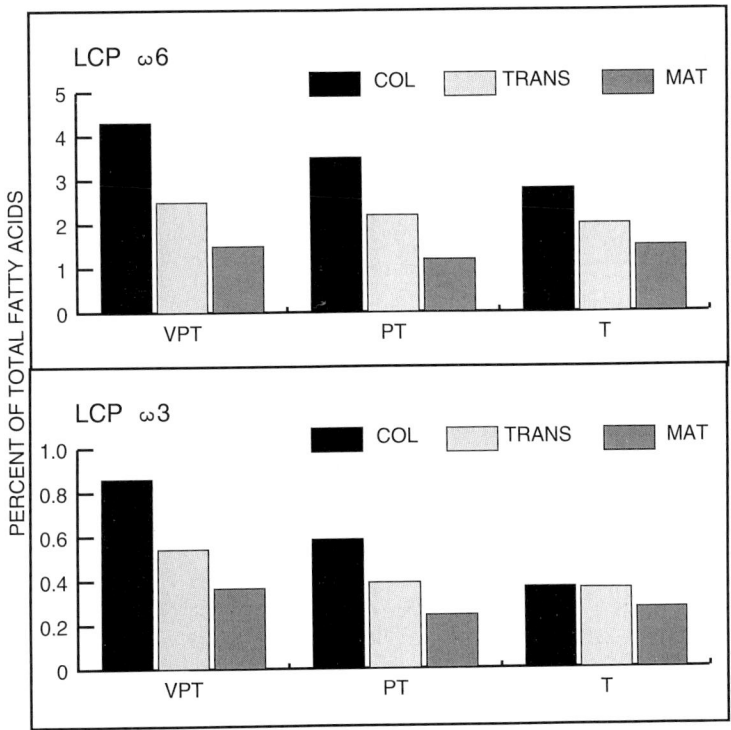

Figure 2. The concentrations of VLC-PUFA's in human milk fat from mothers delivering at 26 to 30 week (VPT), 31 to 36 week (PT) and 37 to 40 week (T) of gestation. COL = colostrum (3 days); TRANS = transitional milk (7 days); MAT = mature milk (21 days). Adapted from Bitman *et al.* (1983).

to the prostaglandins, thromboxanes and prostacyclins. There are only few results on leukotrienes in human milk available, but especially the arachidonic acid derived prostaglandins PGE2 and PGF2alpha have been determined by several authors in human milk.

The very low concentrations for different prostaglandins recently published by Neu et al. (1988) shown in *Table V* indicate "no differences in the milk of mothers delivering prematurely or at term and the concentrations of prostaglandins also remained essentially the same at various stages of lactation" (Neu et al., 1988). These results from Neu et al. (1988) are in contrast to the results of several other authors and especially to the high concentrations of PGE2 published by Chappell et al. (1983) (*see Table V*). This high variance in the prostaglandin concentrations might be due to differences in sample preparation for the radio immuno assay (RIA) as stated by Neu et al. (1988).

Table V. The prostaglandin concentrations [pg/ml] in human milk (term/preterm) during lactation*

Prosta-glandin	Colostrum (1-5d)		Transitional (6-15d)		Mature (≥ 16 d)	
	term	preterm	term	preterm	term	preterm
PGE_2	33 ± 16 (1400 ± 210)**	34 ± 14 3200 ± 730)**	33 ± 33	160 ± 123	7 ± 2 (6920 ± 690)	33 ± 33 3310 ± 660)**
$PGF_{2\alpha}$	14 ± 6	4 ± 2	6 ± 3	7 ± 4	10 ± 3	6 ± 3
$DHKF_{2\alpha}$	85 ± 38	71 ± 20	66 ± 21	148 ± 71	70 ± 16	80 ± 14

* adapted from Neu et al. (1988); C = 3d, T = 7d, M = 21d.
** adapted from Chappell et al. (1983): C = 4d, M = 16d.

In summary, the VLC-PUFA's are found in quite low amounts in human milk, but they are not present in significant amount in infant formulas. VLC-PUFA's in human milk are mainly present in the triglyceride rather than in the phospholipid fraction, although the relative amount of VLC-PUFA's is much higher in the phospholipids. VLC-PUFA's have been shown to be in higher concentrations in preterm than in term human milk. VLC-PUFA's decrease in relative concentration during lactation in term and preterm human milk, nevertheless the absolute quantities seem to remain more or less constant. The VLC-PUFA derived prostaglandins have been shown to be present in relatively very low concentrations in human milk. These results need further evaluation due to analytical problems.

Discussion

Chairman: Thank you very much, Mr Kohn. Any observations and questions on that presentation ?

S. Carlson: A very quick question, what was the linoleic acid concentration in mother diet?

G. Kohn: I think I haven't to check it.

Chairman: Do you have any idea of what the diet the mothers were on at the time?

G. Kohn: Yes, the mothers were on a quite normal Western diet, but we did not check that in detail. The linoleic acid content you asked for was about 10%, it's rather constant.

S. Carlon: I think in the US we have about 15%.

Chairman: And it's going up, isn't it ?

B. Salle: How many mothers did you study for term babies and preterm babies?

G. Kohn: 14 mothers of preterm and also 14 mothers of term.

B. Salle: How did you collect the milk, before or after feeding the babies?

G. Kohn: No, the samples were collected throughout all nursing times and by complete emptying of both breasts, into sterile container. There was an aliquot of 20 ml, just taken from the whole sample.

B. Salle: Did you note the composition of lipid change during suckling time?

G. Kohn: Yes, it changes between fore and hind milk, for sure. Therefore we took the whole sample of all nursing times to the whole day, they were put together and this total sample was analysed.

J. Rey: You didn't speak of the cells in the milk, I think it's very important specially in the colostrum and transitional milk because you know that mother cells diminish very quickly after birth, in the milk. Probably one half of your results can be explained by the different content of cells, especially the very long chain polyunsaturated fatty acids bounds to phospholipids. So I think it could be interesting if you could tell us what is the amount of available very long chain polyunsaturated fatty acids, the part linked with triglycerides, by day, in mother milk. Have you found idea of this and I would like to know if there is any relation between the amount of PUFAs and the diet. Do you try to find a correlation between for example linoleic acid in the milk and the PUFAs ?

G. Kohn: I didn't, but I think the question is rather important. We have to check the lipid content of the cells in human milk, but on the other hand I think the cells do not contain large amounts of triglycerides in the human milk. So the triglyceride content is absolutely the main amount in human milk and so I think that absolutely more than 90% of the very long chain polyunsaturated fatty acids derived from the triglycerides that might not be due to the cells. This question is especially important in relation to the content of eicosanoids because eicosanoids might be a source of prostaglandins; several authors discussed this theme and there is quite a controversy on which part of the total prostaglandins derived from the cells or was produced in the breast.

Chairman: Before I ask Dr Innis to present a question, does anybody in the audience know the answer to the question whether the diet of the mother influences the amount, not of 18:2 18:3 which we know it does, but of the longer chain fatty acids?

B. Koletzko: Linoleic acid and linolenic acid mother dietary intake can determine linoleic and alphalinolenic acid content in maternal milk and this is the reason for the slight difference between Europe and USA. In Europe, it is observed about 10% linoleic acid in human milk, I guess it's the same in Australia, whereas in North America for the last two decades of further increase and now must be obviously closer to 14-15%. However as seen in your slides, this group of mothers who were on a self selected so-called normal Western diet, there was no correlation whatsoever between linoleic acid and the omega 6 and omega 3 LCP content. In other words, linoleic acid intake, linoleic availability does not limit the LCP secretion and we have other data, that I will show tomorrow, but I demonstrate that omega 6 and omega 3 LCP content are closely correlated to each other and that the limiting factor would be the synthesis.

Chairman: Thank you very much and now your question, Dr Innis.

S. Innis: I think your data on long chain polyunsaturated fatty acid composition change in mother milk for preterm and term infant is of special interest. I'd like to raise a question, or a comment in regards of feeding preterm. Usually the preterm babies are not fed immediately after birth. Before we start to feed them, in our unit, we use human milk fortyfier to ensure adequate protein intake so that in preterm we're infact actually feeding mature milk. I think this is very important in trying to optimize the fatty acid status.

Chairman: Yes, thank you, any other comments or questions?

C. Galli: I would like to ask you if you have any data on the vitamin E content, relative to the change in fatty acid in the different stages of lactation?

G. Kohn: We have data but not here, I'm sorry. It is published.

Chairman: Could I just ask one question, you've floated it out, anyone suggesting that the prostaglandins have any biological effect?

G. Kohn: It's quite a controversy, several authors say that the prostaglandins have an effect on the gastro-intestinal tract.

Chairman: They might have effect, but of course they might, has anybody shown that they do have any effect? The speculation is delightful. Is there any evidence? No, nobody going to offer anything? Right, may I thank all the speakers, it has been an interesting session this afternoon, thank you very much indeed.

SESSION IV

Chairman: Sheila INNIS (Canada)

9

Human milk and fatty acids: qualitative aspects

P. SARDA*, D. RIEU**

*Hôpital Saint-Charles, Service de Pédiatrie Néonatale, CHRU de Montpellier,
34059 Montpellier Cedex, France
**Clinique des Enfants Malades, Hôpital Saint-Charles,
300, rue Auguste-Broussonet, 34059 Montpellier Cedex, France

The triacylglycerol content is about 98% of the total lipids. The amounts of phospholipids and sterols vary largely, but these lipid classes have important nutritional consequences in spite of their relatively minor quantities. Phospholipids represent about 1% of the total lipids. However fat globule membrane is a major source of phospholipid, 90% are incorporated in the membrane.

Lipolysis of the triacylglycerol content occurs if the samples are not extracted immediately. Reduction of triacylglycerols is accompanied by an increase in diacylglycerols, monoglycerols and free fatty acids. For instance free fatty acid content is 200 times more important if the samples are stored at $-20°$ and thawed twice.

Human milk fat contains about 10 major fatty acids; therefore, in theory, it would be possible to have 1 000 triacylglycerol species if all the acids were distributed at random. In fact the fatty acid distribution in human milk is asymmetrical and the positional distribution of fatty acids in triacylglycerols differs completely from human and bovine milk or formula.

In human milk, palmitic acid is mainly incorporated in the 2-position; thus 58% of triacylglycerols have a palmitic acid in the 2-position, signifying that 71% of the palmitic acid is on the 2-position. Stearic acid is mainly incorporated in the 1-position and oleic acid in the 1- and 3-positions.

Essential fatty acids are esterified on the 3-positions more randomly. This particular positional distribution of fatty acids in triacylglycerols seems to be specific of the human species.

Few studies have reported an unusual composition of the milk triacylglycerol-structures. *Table I*, concerning a lactating patient with primary type 1 hyperlipidemia,

Table I. Carbon number distribution of milk triacylglycerols from a patient with type 1 hyperlipidemia compared to that of a normal subject (Myher J.J., 1984)

Carbon number	Patient with type 1 hyperlipidemia			Normal subject (13)
	3D	9D	10D	
	(mole %)			
32	0,6	1,8	1,2	–
34	0,7	2,2	1,3	–
36	1,2	4,4	3,6	–
38	1,2	5,1	8,5	–
40	0,8	8,4	14,7	0,9
42	2,5	12,0	17,4	2,1
44	3,0	13,3	14,8	4,7
46	7,1	12,2	13,1	8,2
48	11,2	10,9	8,7	11,6
50	19,8	11,6	7,0	16,8
52	31,5	13,2	6,4	34,0
54	16,7	3,4	2,1	16,7
56	3,5	0,9	0,9	3,6
58	0,5			1,2

represents the gas chromatographic resolution of triacylglycerols on successive days, from day 3 to day 10. As lactation progresses the proportion of the short medium chain triacylglycerols increases. For normal subjects, triacylglycerols with 52 carbons constitute the major fraction (34%). In this patient with hyperlipidemia, only 6% of the triacylglycerols had 52 carbons and the major fraction had 42 carbons at 10 days. Although change in diet can affect the fatty acid composition and consequently the structure, we have little information about the influence of diet on the triacylglycerol structure. In fact fatty acid pattern of breast milk is affected in many situations, for example by diet [vegetarian versus non vegetarian women, the quantity and quality of dietary fat (fish oil, vegetable oil), the quantity of dietary carbohydrates], by maternal weight loss, by the degree of prematurity, or by the stage of lactation. All these modifications probably affect the triacylglycerol structure.

Infant intestinal absorption depends on the characteristics of the structure of ingested triacylglycerols. Hydrolysis of triacylglycerol leads to the production of free fatty acids and 2-monoglycerides, the final result being the transformation of slightly polar lipids to more polar lipids. Palmitic and stearic acids react as non polar lipids and can be solubilized only in the mixed micelles of bile salts and monoglycerides. In human milk 71% of the palmitic acid is esterified at the most favorable 2-position. This explains the better absorption of palmitic acid from human milk as compared with the absorption of this fatty acid from formula.

A particular point must be stressed concerning the structure of fatty acid. The major fatty acids esterified with triacylglycerols are cis fatty acids. However, trans fatty acids deriving from partially hydrogenated food fats consumed by the mother may be important in human milk. Thus trans isomers are present, ranging between 2% and 18% of total fatty acids. The major proportion of trans isomers is 18:1 reflecting the quality of the maternal diet but other trans isomers are detected in human milk as reported on *Table II*. Mean trans fatty acid content in human milk is dependant on ethnic habits. Considerable differences exist between African women who have few trans isomers and European and American women who have the highest levels of trans isomers. Weight loss during lactation also causes an increase in trans fatty acids in milk.

Table II. Trans fatty acids of mature milk in Germany (Koletzko B., 1988)

14:1 t	0,27 ± 0,02
16:1 t	0,50 ± 0,04
18:1 t	3,11 ± 0,15
18:2 tt	0,17 ± 0,01
18:2 ct	0,13 ± 0,01
18:2 tc	0,10 ± 0,01
20:1 t	0,05 ± 0,02

Trans fatty acids are non essential fatty acids. Their intake in diet may have some physiological effects by influencing membrane fluidity, cholesterol metabolism or desaturase activities; in particular trans 18:2 fatty acid depresses activity of delta-6-desaturase. Data showed that isomeric fatty acid in hydrogenated soybean oil inhibited the microsomal delta-6-desaturase activity of liver microsomes isolated from the livers of rats *(Table III)*.

Table III. Effect of dietary fats on rat liver microsomal lipid composition (Mahfouz M.M., 1984)

	Corn oil (%)	Safflower oil (%)	Lard (%)	Hydrogenated fat (%)
Dietary fatty acids				
18:1 *trans*	–	–	0.8	35.1
18:1 *cis*	25.6	76.1	43.5	25.7
18:2 $\omega 6$	61.3	15.2	10.0	15.3
Microsomal fatty acids				
18:1 *trans*	–	–	–	12.8
18:1 *cis*	6.8	15.3	11.8	9.6
18:2 $\omega 6$	15.2	6.1	6.3	10.3
20:4 $\omega 6$	29.8	30.5	29.0	24.6

The influence of cis and trans fatty acids on the composition of the cardiac plasma membrane has been studied (*Table IV*). The animals which received trans fatty acids in their diet incorporated 18:1 trans fatty acid in phosphatidylcholine and phosphatidylethanolamine; this abnormal incorporation may influence micro fluidity of the cardiac membranes.

Table IV. Influence of cis and trans fat on membrane fatty acid composition (Babka B., 1983).

Fatty acid	Phosphatidylcholine			Phosphatidylethanolamine		
	Corn oil (%)	Basal ration (%)	Hydrogenated fat (%)	Corn oil (%)	Basal ration (%)	Hydrogenated fat (%)
18:0	8	8	7	31	33	20
18:1 trans	–	–	3	–	–	8
18:1 cis	16	20	26	7	8	10
18:2	33	30	26	22	14	13

*1% corn oil was added to the basal corn/soybean ration; 10% corn oil or 9% hydrogenated soy oil (50% trans acids) was added to the basal ration, respectively.

The amount of total cholesterol in human milk has been reported as ranging from 200 to more than 1 130 mg per 100 g of lipid. But variations of 30% were noted in the same woman, from month to month. The large differences in the quantities of cholesterol found by authors can probably be attributed to the use of non specific methods of determination. Therefore phytosterols, lanosterols and desmosterols could overestimate the cholesterol content of milk.

Most of the cholesterol present in human milk exists as free cholesterol. A minor percentage (10 to 20%) exists in the esterified form, particularly with the long chain fatty acids. Cholesterol content is higher in colostrum (over 20 mg per dl), but this amount decreases exponentially during lactation. In mature milk, total cholesterol, cholesteryl esters and free cholesterol are stable. *Table V* shows the stability of cholesterol levels throughout 3 to 56 weeks of lactation.

Table V. Amount of cholesterol in human milk during lactation (Bitman J., 1986).

Sample	Lactation		Total cholesterol (mg/dl)	Cholesteryl ester (mg/dl)	Percent ester
	Stage	Days			
1	Colostrum	3	23.70	4.22	17.8
2	Colostrum	4	22.80	5.61	24.6
3	Transitional	10	13.40	1.88	14.0
4	Mature	21	9.60	1.26	13.1
5	Mature	135	8.00	0.72	9.0
6	Mature	150	5.90	0.59	10.0
7	Mature	390	7.60	1.10	14.5

The effects of diet on the cholesterol and phytosterol in human milk are presented on *Table VI*. Cholesterol in milk is not correlated with dietary cholesterol. But a large amount in dietary phytosterol increased the amount of phytosterol in milk, from 17 mg to 220 mg per 100 g of fat.

Table VI. Effects of dietary cholesterol, phytosterol and polyunsaturate/saturate ratio on human milk sterol (Mellies M.J., 1978)

Milk component	Maternal *ad lib* diet (P/S 0.53) (mg/100 g fat)	Low cholesterol/high phytosterol diet (P/S 1.8) (mg/100 g fat)	High cholesterol/flow phytosterol diet (P/S 0.12) (mg/100 g fat)
Cholesterol	240 ± 40	250 ± 10	250 ± 20
Phytosterol	17 ± 3	220 ± 30	70 ± 10
Dietary cholesterol	450 ± 30	130 ± 5	460 ± 90
Dietary phytosterol	23 ± 8	790 ± 17	80 ± 1
Total fat (%)	3.58 ± 0.56	2.69 ± 0.17	2.66 ± 0.16

Fatty acid composition of the cholesteryl esters in human colostrum is presented on *Table VII*. The concentration of saturated fatty acids with less than 16 carbons is lower in preterm than in term colostrum (23% versus 35%). On the other hand, the concentration of long chain unsaturated fatty acids was higher in preterm colostrum. In mature milk (*Table VIII*), there are few differences between the fatty acids in cholesteryl esters of preterm and term milk. During lactation, major changes between colostrum and mature milk are the reduction of palmitic acid and an increase in the proportion of linoleic acid from 20% to 32%.

Table VII. Comparison of the fatty acid composition of the cholesteryl esters in human colostrum (Bitman J., 1986)

Fatty acid	Preterm (%)	Term (%)
≤ 16:0	23	35
18:1	31.5 ± 2.7	28.9 ± 6.5
18:2	24.0 ± 2.3	21.3 ± 8.4
18:3	1.3 ± 0.4	0.5 ± 0.5
20:3	1.5 ± 0.4	0.4 ± 0.4
20:4	2.8 ± 0.4	0.9 ± 0.9

Trans fatty acids are found in cholesteryl esters. Trans 18:1 isomer is the major trans fatty acid.

Phospholipids represent about 1% of the total lipids. Phosphatidylcholine, phosphatidylethanolamine and sphyngomyelin are the principal components in human milk (*Table IX*). Milk phospholipids from term babies exhibited a continuous decrease

Table VIII. Comparison of the fatty acid composition of the cholesteryl esters in mature milk (Bitman J., 1986)

Fatty acid	Preterm (%)	Term (%)
≤ 16:0	17	15
18:1	30 ±2.5	34.4±2.8
18:2	32.8±2.3	31.2±2.7
18:3	2.0±0.4	1.6±0.4
20:3	1.0±0.2	0.4±0.1
20:4	1.8±0.4	1.0±0.4

Table IX. Phospholipid class distribution during lactation (Harzer G., 1983)

Phospholipids	Percentage of total phospholipid on day							
	1	3	5	8	15	22	29	36
Sphingomyelin	28.3	29.3	29.2	29.9	30.9	31.1	32.9	32.4
Phosphatidylcholine	35.2	29.2	31.3	29.0	27.4	26.7	25.2	24.9
Phosphatidylserine	9.2	12.9	8.4	8.3	9.4	8.5	9.6	9.3
Phosphatidylinositol	5.1	6.5	4.8	5.1	5.2	5.0	5.4	5.4
Phosphatidylethanolamine	22.3	26.8	26.3	28.0	27.9	28.5	26.5	27.7

during lactation; the concentration decreases from colostrum (1 %) to mature milk (0,5 %). Preterm milk phospholipids are higher than those of term milk, but an identical decrease is observed during lactation.

During lactation phospholipid class distribution is relatively stable. This is not surprising since the phospholipids of human milk are issued from the globule membrane and thus from the secretory plasma membrane of the mammary gland which is identical at all stages of lactation. This distribution is also identical with the distribution found in other species such as cow, sheep, pig, camel, etc. Some studies have reported the changes of the composition of fatty acids in the different phospholipid class with lactation, but the results are sometimes very discordant. The most constant change is an increase of the linoleic acid in all phospholipid classes, as lactation progressed from colostrum to mature milk.

Table X shows the usual distribution of fatty acids such as phosphatidylcholine and phosphatidylethanolamine; the saturated fatty acids are essentially and normally at the 1-position and the polyunsaturated fatty acids at the 2-position. Trans fatty acids are also present (2,5 % to 3,6 %).

Gibson demonstrated a lack of correlation between linoleic and arachidonic acid in human milk. Other authors also reported the same lack of correlation between linolenic acid and omega 3 long chain polyunsaturated fatty acids. The very long chain polyunsaturated fatty acid content of human milk does not appear to be closely related to maternal diet, probably because these fatty acids are essentially in the phospholipids and thus in the globule membrane.

Table X. Distribution of fatty acids as phosphatidylcholine and phosphatidylethanolamine in human milk (Hundreiser K.E., 1983)

Fatty acid	Phosphatidylcholine (wt %)			Phosphatidylethanolamine (wt %)		
	sn-1	sn-2[b]	Total	sn-1	sn-2[b]	Total
10:0	1.33± 0.90	0.00	0.60±0.61	2.56± 2.23	0.00	1.01±1.12
12:0	2.16± 1.65	0.34	1.25±1.14	1.49± 0.76	0.27	0.88±0.94
14:0	6.09± 3.22	0.93	3.51±2.40	4.28± 2.59	0.00	1.97±1.40
16:0	31.71±11.17	19.79	25.75±7.06	22.52± 9.86	0.00	11.17±6.31
16:1	4.85± 5.35	4.11	4.48±4.98	7.29± 5.73	0.11	3.70±3.96
18:0	16.31±10.88	23.05	19.68±9.19	23.30±14.37	30.46	26.88±8.99
trans-18:1	1.92± 0.84	3.12	2.52±0.96	3.03± 2.00	4.27	3.65±3.22
cis-18:1	20.08± 9.93	7.78	13.93±3.21	19.73± 6.08	19.95	19.84±6.40
18:2	5.80± 5.83	25.54	15.67±7.70	4.34± 2.66	23.00	13.67±8.88
18:3 + 20:1	1.13± 0.62	0.95	1.04±0.64	1.12± 0.77	3.53	2.47±1.06
22:0	0.45± 0.39	1.25	0.85±0.42	0.63± 0.46	1.51	1.07±0.75
20:3	0.20± 0.09	0.14	0.17±0.14	0.76± 0.82	0.08	0.42±0.35
20:4	0.71± 0.81	2.11	1.41±0.66	0.67± 0.55	11.53	6.10±4.84
20:5	0.62± 0.25	6.42	3.52±4.24	tr	2.44	1.22±0.96
22:6	tr	2.34	1.17±1.24	tr	1.68	0.84±1.29

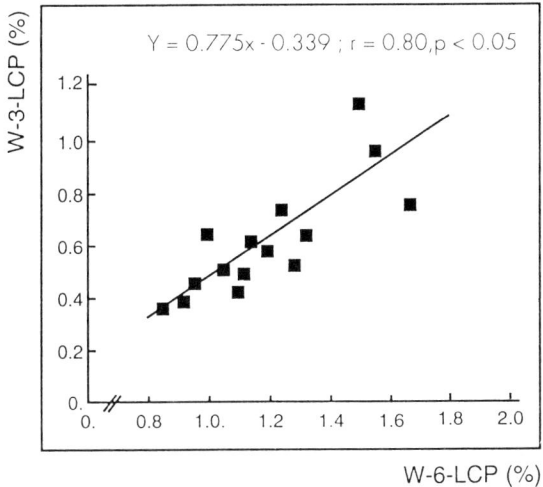

Figure 1. Correlation of LCPU fatty acid content of the ω3 and the ω6 series in human milk lipids (Koletzko B., 1988).

Koletzko (*figure 1*) showed that the omega-3 long chain polyunsaturated fatty acids were significantly correlated to the omega-6 long chain polyunsaturated fatty acids. This result suggests that there are individual differences in the capacity of maternal elongase/desaturase activity. Some babies may have a better supply than others.

Discussion

Chairman: Any questions from the floor? Maybe I can start with a question. I was interested in your data on the phytosterols in milk. Are these sterols well absorbed by the nursing infant?

P. Sarda: I don't know exactly but I think phytosterols are not absorbed by intestinal tract.

A. Crastes de Paulet: Phytosterols are poorly absorbed. There is a competition between the absorption of phytosterols and cholesterol, but when the supply of phytosterol is in a normal range, the level of phytosterols in the plasma is very low but of course you must show data showing the very high level of phytosterol in the milk, but I suppose that it was megadose.

Chairman: Perhaps I could follow that with a question on milk formula, are there plant sterols in the lipids used in infant formula?

J.M. Bourre: I was interested by the occurrence of trans isomers in the milk, as you mentioned. As you probably know a high amount of energy has been used to avoid to get the right technique to prove that this trans fatty acid could be eventually toxic.

As they are present in the milk, they could be present also in the foetus, or in the newborn, in the tissues. So what is the relationship between the amount of trans isomers eaten by the mother, the amount found in the blood and the amount found in the milk. Do you have any data on this?

P. Sarda: I think there is a relation but I don't know studies with augmentation of trans fatty acid in the diet and correspondence in the newborn. But in countries where trans fatty acids are high in the diet you find a large quantity in the milk and in the foetus, in the newborn too. The largest quantities are found in the USA, in Canada.

J.M. Bourre: Yes, I am wondering if you can get some barrier in the production of the milk, avoiding to get iatrogenic trans isomers in the milk.

P. Sarda: I don't know, I don't know if Koletzko was working on trans fatty acid.

B. Koletzko: I think it has been actually shown that trans fatty acid content in milk very much depends on trans fatty acid mother diet. We have done studies which are published, to compare trans fatty acid content of mothers from Africa, which have of course a very low dietary intake of trans isomers and don't consume hydrogenated fats, with mothers from Germany. There was a tremendous difference in the trans fatty acid content reflecting the difference in diet and also the difference between most European countries and especially the USA reflects dietary differences.

J. Rey: In a project of directives of the EEC, the amount of trans fatty acid will be limited to a certain percent. I would like to add that the preferential localisation of palmitic acid in the 2-position is not specific of humans, it's also observed in sow milk and lard, and 20 years ago Nestle Company tried to manufacture a product with lard fat, instead of milk fat, but it's too expensive and many problems arise at the using of pork in the preparation of formula.

O. Hernell: I would like to make a comment about the importance of this 2-position. It is really important. When you compare the absorption of fat with the same fatty acid in position 2, you would expect to find the same type of absorption for stearic acid for example. However you don't have a better absorption of stearic acid. There is something special going on with palmitic acid and it's probably not only the 2-position.

P. Sarda: Yes, it's probably true. But in human milk you have many things which conduct to a better absorption probably calcium, protein and it's not only the position on the triglyceride.

Chairman: Is there any other question ? So I can thank Dr Sarda.

10

Human milk nucleotides and essential fatty acid metabolism during early life

M.L. PITA

Universidad de Granada, Departamento de Bioquimica y Biologica Molecular, Facultad de Ciencias, 18071 Granada, Spain

First of all I wish to thank Mr Ghisolfi and Dr Putet for their kind invitation to this meeting. Thank you very much.

As we all know, nucleotides play important roles for many cellular functions. They act as precursors for nucleic acids synthesis but they are also implicated in cell metabolism as enzyme regulators, allosteric effectors and cell messengers. Nucleic acids and nucleotides are constantly being formed and degraded, especially in tissues with high turnover rates such as intestinal mucosa, skin or white and red blood cells. Purine and pyrimidine nucleotides can be formed in most tissues by *de novo* synthesis from amino acids, carbon dioxide and other precursors. Alternatively, nucleotides can be reconstituted via the salvage pathway using free bases derived either from dietary nucleotides or from the catabolism of nucleic acids. There is evidence that some tissues such as lymphocytes or enterocytes present a limited activity or a limited capacity for the *de novo* synthesis of purine and pyrimidine nucleotides and preferentially utilize preformed bases *via* the salvage pathway. For these tissues an adequate supply of exogenous nucleotides can be important for optimal function.

Some metabolic and physiologic effects of dietary nucleotides have been described in the last years. For example, intestinal iron absorption is enhanced in the presence of inosine and it has also been demonstrated that human milk nucleotides stimulate both *in vivo* and *in vitro* growth of intestinal bifidobacteria thus limiting the proliferation of other microorganisms such as enterobacteria or lactobacilli. Dietary nucleotides have also been related to cell mediated immunity. They stimulate the lymphoproliferative response to alloantigens, the phagocytic activity of macrophages and the delayed cutaneous hypersensitivity. Finally, recent studies have demonstrated that exogenous nucleotides inhibit liver injury after galactosamin administration and stimulate *in vitro* proliferation of hepatocytes and hepatocarcinoma cells.

Nucleotides are present in foods mainly in the form of nucleoproteins. After digestion, a mix of nucleotides and free bases are absorbed via the intestinal mucosa. However, soluble nucleotides have been found in milk from various mammals, contributing up to 20% of the non-protein nitrogen. In human milk acid soluble nucleotides were described for the first time about 30 years ago. Since this time, at least 13 different free nucleotides have been identified in human milk.

The nucleotide profile of human milk and cow milk is shown in *Table I*. We can see that human milk contains relatively high concentrations of cytidine, uridine and adenosine nucleotides and low levels of guanosine and inosine derivatives. Conversely, cow milk only contains low levels of cytidine and adenosine nucleotides but it contains a high concentration of orotate which is practically absent in human milk.

Table I. Nucleotide composition of human milk, cow milk and levels of nucleotides added to the adapted milk formula (NMF)

	Human milk (µmoles/dl)	Cow milk (µmoles/dl)	NMF (mg/100g)
CMP	1.97 ± 0.04	3.32 ± 0.24	1.12
AMP	2.09 ± 0.11	2.75 ± 0.14	1.32
GMP	0.16 ± 0.03	n.d.	1.49
UMP	1.12 ± 0.07	n.d.	3.42
Orotate	n.d.	36.73 ± 2.23	–
IMP	–	–	0.45

The results are mean ± SEM. n.d. = not detected

In relation to these marked differences between the nucleotide content in human milk and cow milk, our research group has investigated the possible influence of dietary nucleotides on lipid metabolism in newborns during postnatal development. Initially, in our first study, we exclusively analysed the total fatty acid composition of plasma in term newborn infants fed human milk, a standard milk formula or the same standard milk formula supplemented with nucleotides at levels similar to those found in human milk. *Table I* shows the nucleotides added to this formula (CMP, AMP, GMP, UMP, IMP). Samples were obtained at birth, after one week and after four weeks of life. I am going to comment only the modifications of polyunsaturated fatty acids since saturated and monounsaturated fatty acids were mostly unaffected by diet.

Table II shows the changes of linoleic acid in the plasma of newborn infants at birth, after one week and after four weeks of life. Infants were fed human milk, the milk formula and the nucleotide supplemented milk formula. We can see that after one month of life the two groups of infants fed formula presented a higher concentration of linoleic acid in plasma as compared to the human milk fed infants. However, as we can see, the dihomo-γ-linolenic acid was markedly decreased at one month of life in infants fed exclusively the standard milk formula and the other two groups of infants showed similar values for this fatty acid. Arachidonic acid showed the same decrease in the group of infants fed a standard milk formula and again

Table II. Plasma concentrations of linoleic acid, dihomo-γ-linolenic acid and arachidonic acid in term infants fed HM, MF and NMF during the first month of life

Fatty acids	6-8 h	Diet	Time of delivery	
			1 week	4 weeks
18: 2 n–6	12.8 ± 1.0	HM	13.4 ± 0.8	17.8 ± 1.7
		MF	18.1 ± 0.1[a]	25.8 ± 1.0[ab]
		NMF	16.8 ± 1.0[a]	20.2 ± 1.9[a]
20: 3 n–6	0.8 ± 0.2	HM	1.5 ± 0.1	2.1 ± 0.2
		MF	1.1 ± 0.2	1.5 ± 0.2
		NMF	1.7 ± 0.3	2.4 ± 0.3
20: 4 n–6	19.8 ± 1.2	HM	11.8 ± 1.3	7.1 ± 1.3
		MF	10.0 ± 1.3[a]	5.6 ± 0.9[ab]
		NMF	8.9 ± 0.9[a]	8.3 ± 0.4

The results are mean percentages ± SEM. HM: infant group fed human milk. MF: infant group fed milk formula. NMF: infant group fed nucleotide supplemented formula. a $p > 0.05$ versus HM; b $p > 0.05$ versus NMF.

the other two groups of infants fed human milk and the nucleotide supplemented milk formula showed similar values for this fatty acid. When we determined the fatty acid profile of each plasma lipid fraction in the same experimental conditions we found the same modifications. In plasma phospholipids, which is the most unsaturated plasma lipid fraction, we found again a high level of linoleic acid in the two groups of infants fed formulas and a decrease in arachidonic acid, the major metabolite of linoleic acid, in infants fed the standard milk formula (*Table III*). α-linolenic acid was unaffected by diet but its major metabolite docosahexaenoic acid was decreased in infants fed a standard milk formula. Human milk fed infants showed higher levels for this fatty acid and the infants fed nucleotide supplemented formula showed intermediate values for this fatty acid.

We know that for essential fatty acids, the conversion to longer metabolites depends on elongation and desaturation processes. It has been suggested that in newborn infants, Δ6 and Δ5-desaturases present a limited activity and there is also a growing evidence that a high supply of linoleic acid inhibits the activity of both acylCoA desaturases. So the lower levels of plasma polyunsaturated fatty acids found in our study in infants fed the standard milk formula could be due to the impairment of desaturase activities by linoleic acid since milk formulas used in our study contained about 24% of this fatty acid. Additionally, we know that human milk contains relatively high amounts of preformed polyunsaturated fatty acids, thus contributing to increase the plasma polyunsaturated fatty acids in infants fed human milk. However, the only difference found between the two milk formulas used in our study was their nucleotide content. So we have speculated with the possibility that dietary nucleotides are influencing the enterocyte or hepatocyte polyunsaturated fatty acid synthesis in newborn infants, perhaps through an enhancement of desaturase activities. This hypothesis is supported by the lower archidonic to linoleic acid ratio found

Table III. Linoleic acid, α-linolenic acid, arachidonic acid and docosahexaenoic acid levels of plasma phospholipids in term infants fed HM, MF or NMF during the first month of life

Fatty acids	Diet	Time of delivery	
		1 week	4 weeks
18:2 n–6	HM	12.4 ± 1.4	13.5 ± 1.0
	MF	18.8 ± 1.1[a]	21.8 ± 0.7[a]
	NMF	19.3 ± 0.8[a]	26.6 ± 1.2[ab]
18:3 n–3	HM	0.8 ± 0.5	0.3 ± 0.1
	MF	0.7 ± 0.4	0.4 ± 0.1
	NMF	0.3 ± 0.1	0.3 ± 0.0
20:4 n–6	HM	12.4 ± 1.4	8.2 ± 1.2
	MF	8.7 ± 0.7[a]	4.4 ± 0.5[a]
	NMF	10.8 ± 0.5[b]	6.6 ± 0.7[ab]
22:6 n–3	HM	2.7 ± 0.3	1.9 ± 0.4
	MF	1.8 ± 0.2[a]	0.4 ± 0.1[a]
	NMF	2.4 ± 0.2[b]	0.9 ± 0.2[ab]

The results are mean percentages ± SEM. HM: infant group fed human milk. MF: infant group fed milk formula. NMF: infant group fed nucleotide supplemented milk formula. a $p < 0.05$ versus HM; b $p < 0.05$ versus MF.

after one month of life in infants fed the standard milk formula as compared to those fed human milk and nucleotide supplemented milk formula.

Using the same study protocol we have also demonstrated that dietary nucleotides also affect the fatty acid composition of erythrocyte membrane phospholipids both in term and preterm infants. In term infants we have determined the fatty acid profile of the four major phospholipid fractions found in cell membranes, phosphatidylcholine, phosphatidylethanolamine, phosphatidylserine and sphyngomyelin. We have found, after one month of life, that long chain polyunsaturated fatty acids from n–6 series (PUFA n–6 > 18C) were decreased in infants fed a standard milk formula as compared to the other studied groups, especially in phosphatidylethanolamine which is the most unsaturated phospholipid fraction found in membranes (*Table IV*). Polyunsaturated fatty acids of n–3 series (PUFA n–3 > 18C) were also decreased in infants fed the standard milk formula and again phosphatidylethanolamine showed the most marked decrease for these fatty acids.

In preterm infants we have determined the total fatty acid composition of red blood cell membrane phospholipids; we have also found, at one month of life, a decrease of polyunsaturated fatty acids on n–6 and n–3 series in infants fed a standard milk formula. However, in this study, differences between the three studied groups were less marked than in the study performed with term infants.

All these changes found in fatty acid composition of cell membranes induced by dietary nucleotides probably modify lipid metabolism in newborn infants. For

Table IV. Long chain polyunsaturated fatty acids of the n–6 and n–3 series or erythrocyte membrane fractions in newborn infants fed HM, MF or NMF at 30 days of life

	Diet	Erythrocyte membrane fractions			
		PE	PC	PS	SM
n–6 PUFA > 18C	HM	19.7 ± 2.4	6.2 ± 1.0	13.9 ± 2.2	3.8 ± 1.1
	MF	9.0 ± 2.3[a]	3.8 ± 1.2	8.4 ± 2.5	1.1 ± 0.3[a]
	NMF	20.3 ± 2.3[b]	5.4 ± 0.7	12.9 ± 1.9	1.6 ± 0.4
n–3 PUFA > 18C	HM	5.3 ± 0.9	0.8 ± 0.3	3.0 ± 1.0	0.9 ± 0.5
	MF	1.2 ± 0.5[a]	0.5 ± 0.1	1.6 ± 0.7	n.d.
	NMF	3.5 ± 0.9	0.6 ± 0.2	2.3 ± 0.8	n.d.

The results are mean percentages ± SEM. HM: infant group fed human milk. MF: infant group fed milk formula. NMF: infant group fed nucleotide supplemented milk formula. PE: phosphatidylethanolamine. PC: phosphatidylcholine. PS: phosphatidylserine. SM: sphyngomyelin. a $p < 0.05$ versus HM; b $p < 0.05$ versus MF. n.d.: not detected.

example, the higher values found for polyunsaturated fatty acids in infants fed diets with relatively high concentration of nucleotides could modify the availability of precursors for eicosanoid synthesis. Moreover, the lower value found for PUFA n–6 to PUFA n–3 ratio in infants fed human milk or nucleotide supplemented milk formula could improve the synthesis of prostaglandins, thromboxanes and leucotrienes derived from eicosapentaenoic acid, thus limiting inflammatory processes and platelet aggregation. In the other hand, a major availability of polyunsaturated fatty acids of n–3 series in newborn infants and especially in preterm infants could also favour the functionality of some tissues such as central nervous system or retina where these fatty acids and especially docosahexaenoic acid are present in high concentrations.

Changes induced by dietary nucleotides could also modify the degree of desaturation of cell membranes, at least of erythrocyte membrane. Preterm infants fed the standard milk formula showed a decrease of unsaturation index at one month of life as compared to the other studied groups, and also a slight increase in cholesterol to phospholipid molar ratio in this membrane (*Table V*). As a consequence, erythrocyte membrane fluidity might be decreased in these conditions, thus affecting the normal functionality of erythrocytes.

Table V. Unsaturation index (UNID) and cholesterol/phosphorus molar ratio (C/P) in erythrocyte membrane phospholipids of preterm infants fed HM, MF or NMF at 30 days of life

	HM	MF	NMF
UNID	149 ± 5	116 ± 4[a]	131 ± 8
C/P	0.87 ± 0.12	1.26 ± 0.18[a]	0.87 ± 0.11

The results are mean ± SEM. HM: infant group fed human milk. MF: infant group fed milk formula. NMF: infant group fed nucleotide supplemented milk formula. a $p < 0.05$ versus HM.

All these results suggest that dietary nucleotides are influencing the *in vivo* conversion of essential fatty acids to its longer metabolites during early life. Enterocytes or liver desaturases may be either activated or induced by these compounds. Although the nutritional significance of dietary nucleotides for newborn infants needs further investigation, we can conclude that it could be convenient for newborn infants, and especially for preterm infants, to receive an adequate intake of nucleotides, either from human milk or from milk formulas spplemented with these compounds.

Discussion

Chairman: Thank you Dr Pita, are there any questions?

S. Carlson: I have a question about the fatty acid composition of formula, what did you show in the fatty acid composition of formula, that's the same composition you had both in the nucleotide supplemented and non-supplemented formulas?

M.L. Pita: The fat for the milk formula? It's different for formulas for term infants and for preterm infants. In term infants the fat was a mix of butter fat, cornoil, soya and MCT from coconut oil. For preterm infants, we substituted the cornoil for olive oil, so preterm infants in formula have butter fat, soya, MCT and olive oil, a high level of olive oil. And I don't remember the percentage of soya 20%, I don't remember the exact level. The percentage of alphalinolenic acid in formulas was 1.9% for term infants and 1.3% for preterm infants, I think.

S. Carlson: If the alphalinolenic acid is really about 2% of the total fatty acid amount, compared to our results, docosahexaenoic acid you found in these formula fed infants seems to be extremely low?

M.L. Pita: That's what I found, I don't know why.

C. Galli: Have you any information on the effects of the nucleotides on lipoprotein profiles because it has been shown that nucleotides can affect the secretion of the lipoprotein.

M.L. Pita: We have a study by our research group that has demonstrated that dietary nucleotide intake stimulates the synthesis HDL lipoproteins, only the HDL but I have no other study.

J. Rey: Do you know if nucleotides have an effect on the red cell membrane?

M.L. Pita: Directly on the membrane? I don't know.

J. Rey: The effect on long chain fatty acids could be secondary to a change in the membrane.

M.L. Pita: I don't know.

Chairman: Your data could be quite provocative. Would you think that the effect of the nucleotides on the desaturation system could be different in function of organs?

M.L. Pita: We think that the effect of dietary nucleotides is most at the level of the enterocyte than at the liver.

Chairman: Have you any idea of what proportion of HDL are synthesised by the liver?

M.L. Pita : I have no data.

Chairman: If there aren't any other questions I thank you again for a very nice talk.

SESSION V

Chairman: Jean-Marie BOURRE (France)

11

Docosahexaenoate (DHA) and eicosapentaenoate (EPA) supplementation of preterm (PT) infants: effects on RBC and plasma N-3 and visual acuity

S.E. CARLSON, R.J. COOKE, J.M. PEEPLES, S.H. WERKMAN, E.A. TOLLEY

College of Medicine, Department of Pediatrics, 853 Jefferson Avenue, Memphis, TN 38163, USA

I want to thank Dr Ghisolfi, Dr Putet, and Milupa Company for inviting me. My talk today will be about the biochemical and functional aspects of docosahexaenoic acid (DHA) and eicosapentaenoic acid (EPA) supplementation of preterm infants. Rather than speaking about any of our past studies, I am going to talk about one that is in progress at the moment. This study has been going on for over two years. Dr Richard Cooke is the neonatologist on this project. Jeannie Peeples and Susan Werkman are the technician and research nurses, and Dr Tolley is our biostatistician.

As a quick background, retinal and brain grey matter phospholipids are highly enriched in docosahexaenoic acid. Most of this docosahexaenoic acid accumulates between 26 and 40 weeks' post-conceptional age. We know this from Dr Clandinin and co-workers' data. Human milk contains both docosahexaenoic and its precursor linolenic acid. Infants fed linolenic acid as the only source of n–3 fatty acid have large postnatal declines in phospholipid docosahexaenoic compared to infants fed human milk. Like human milk feeding, formulas containing a marine oil source of EPA and DHA will also prevent declines in red blood cell DHA. We published this three years ago in *Pediatric Research*. Failure to accumulate docosahexaenoic acid during development in the animal models has resulted in deficits in visual acuity, retinal physiology, and cognitive function. We have seen some of that data from the rat functional model. Preterm infants may risk poor retinal and neural DHA accumulation because of early delivery and feeds without docosahexaenoic acid. We wanted to compare infants receiving docosahexaenoic acid with those whom we postulated would accumulate inadequate docosahexaenoic acid from standard formula. The functions we have looked at are visual acuity and cognitive function. Data from Neuringer and Connor showed that young monkeys from mothers which were fed soybean oil during gestation have relatively high docosahexaenoic acid in plasma phospholipid at birth. When the mothers were fed safflower oil, the infant monkeys have a much lower level at the time they were born. The level falls even further when they are continued on the safflower oil diet. By the time these infant monkeys were four weeks of age, they already had poorer visual acuity and that continued with time. The question we are trying to answer is: Do preterm infants accumulate sufficient DHA? We do not set out to make infants n–3 deficient, and, in fact, we give them rather high levels of linolenic acid. In the study that I will discuss today, we provided linolenic acid as 3% of total fatty acids in the preterm formula, and then these babies were switched to a 5% linolenic acid formulation when they were 1800 grams. They were continued on the last formula for at least six months. Today I am only presenting preliminary data to six months.

One might think these babies would not become as n–3 deficient as infant monkeys because the monkeys receive soybean oil which contains linolenic acid. These monkeys had much higher levels of DHA than those fed safflower oil. On the other hand, preterm infants have a more limited retinal and neural n–3 accumulation at birth than term infants, and term human infants have less than the term monkeys. So, initially, preterm human infants may be more deficient than term infant monkeys with greater needs for DHA accumulation. Here the acuity norms for human infants are superimposed on those of monkeys of the same ages. The 4-week-old infant sees very poorly compared to a 4-week-old monkey. The acuity of both human and monkey infants improves with time.

We started this study with several questions. (1) How do phospholipid fatty acids, especially DHA, EPA, and AA, change when preterm infants receive linolenic acid as 3%-5% of their fatty acids through much of infancy? (2) How do these same fatty acids change in infancy when additional long chain n–3, that is EPA and DHA, is consumed in the formula? (3) Would phospholipid EPA or DHA relate to the acuity or cognitive function of these babies?

Infants were enrolled according to an IRB protocol and randomized to receive or not receive very long chain n–3 supplementation (.2% DHA and .3% EPA) of total fatty acids. Blood samples were obtained at enrollment and again at term, 48, 57, and 68 weeks' postconception. Plasma and red blood cell phospholipid fatty acids were determined on each sample by capillary gas liquid chromatography.

Visual acuity was measured using the Teller acuity card procedure beginning at term and thereafter at each return visit. Infants' acuity is determined at a specific distance from black and white cards made with stripes of specific widths. Determinations of acuity were made without knowledge of the infants' diet. The acuity data were analyzed by analysis of variance (formula and time), and stepwise regression including the perinatal, neonatal, and biochemical variables collected on these babies. These variables include hours of oxygen (log), hours of mechanical ventilatory support (log), and maternal gravida.

Table I provides the characteristics of the infants studied to date. The control and n–3 supplemented groups were statistically the same for all parameters. The criteria for enrollment were: (1) an energy intake of greater than 110 Kcal per kg per day

Table I. Characteristics of study population

	Control	N-3 Supplemented
Number of infants	29	30
Birthweight (g)	1118 ± 43	1172 ± 32
Enrollment weight (g)	1329 ± 33	1339 ± 21
Age at enrollment (d)	25 ± 2	22 ± 2
Gestation age (wks)	29.6 ± 0.4	29.8 ± 0.3
Apgar Score (5 min)	7.0 ± 0.3	7.2 ± 0.3
Ventilator (hrs)	66 ± 22	35 ± 13
Oxygen (total hrs)	156 ± 453	157 ± 62
Maternal age (yrs)	22.0 ± 1	23.4 ± 1
Gravida	2.5 ± 0.3	2.5 ± 0.3

of preterm formula; (2) a birth weight between 750-1350 grams with a gestational age of less than 32 weeks; (3) absence of need for mechanical ventilation at the time of enrollment; (4) an oxygen requirement less than 25% under hood at enrollment; (5) a negative history for IVH/PVH greater than grade 2 because we wanted to do cognitive function tests on these infants; (6) a negative history of retinopathy of prematurity greater than grade 1 (an ophthalmologist examined retinas of all infants); (7) a negative history of necrotizing enterocolitis requiring surgical resection; and (8) a negative history of maternal substance abuse. At the time of enrollment, plasma phospholipid DHA was intermediate between that reported for n-3 deficient and sufficient monkey infants. The plasma phospholipid DHA of unsupplemented infants did not change with time, but those who received very long chain n-3 supplementation showed an increase in DHA which plateaued somewhere around 48 weeks' postconception.

Table II shows the effect of time and n-3 supplementation on red blood cell phosphatidylethanolamine (PE), EPA, and DHA. At enrollment the mean post-conceptional age was 33 weeks. At that time these babies had a relatively high DHA concentration in PE. From previous studies, we know that cord blood levels are consistently much higher than this, in the range of 9%-10% DHA. By 38 weeks' postconception (term), there is a drop in PE DHA in the control group. In contrast to Dr Sheila Innis's data, which you just saw, I should point out that these babies have now been on term formula with or without very long chain n-3 fatty acids for something like three weeks, and the term formula has a higher linoleic acid than the preterm formula. In other words, there is a decrease by five weeks after enrollment, but there has been a diet change in between. The n-3 supplemented infants show a non-significant decline here. By 48 weeks, DHA has dropped even further in controls, and supplemented infants have stabilized at around 7%. The controls dropped further by five weeks. By 69 weeks, DHA is twofold higher in the PE of the supplemented compared to unsupplemented babies. Keep in mind that both groups are receiving a formula with 5% linolenic acid. EPA does not change in control infants but goes up in the supplemented infants.

The effect of time and n-3 supplementation on acuity is shown in *Table III*. The analysis includes 166 acuity observations from 56 subjects. Because the study is

Table II. Effect of time and n–3 supplementation on red blood cell phosphatidylethanolamine (PE) docosahexaenoate (DHA) and eicosapentaenoate (EPA)

Postconception (wks)	DHA		EPA	
	Control	N–3 Supp	Control	N–Supp
33	7.0	6.9	0.42	0.41
38	5.1	6.6	0.47	1.26
48	4.1	7.3	0.44	1.76
57	3.9	7.5	0.55	2.04
68	3.4	7.3	0.42	2.16
ANOVA: Formula	$P < 0.0001$		$P < 0.0001$	
Time	$P < 0.0001$		$P < 0.0001$	

still in progress, some of these babies have observations at each time to six months of age while others have been studied only at term. These acuity data are in Snellen equivalents which become smaller as acuity becomes better. You can see that there is a significant effect of both time and very long n–3 supplementation on acuity.

Table III. Effect of time and n–3 supplementation on acuity (Snellen equivalents, partial analysis with 56 subjects, 166 acuity observations)

Postconception (wks)	Acuity	
	Control	N–3 Supplemented
33	Not done	Not done
38	697	599
48	274	175
57	118	95
68	80	61
ANOVA: Formula	$P < 0.007$	
Time	$P < 0.0001$	

I do not want you to get the idea that the control infants have poor vision. In fact, the control infants have acuities like the mean for the Teller acuity norms. The effect of very long n–3 supplementation is an actual enhancement of acuity above the norm. Supplemented infants actually had a mean acuity at six months equivalent to the mean for 15-month-old infants.

In addition to looking at the mean acuities for the groups, we looked at the determinants of acuity at these study ages. Stepwise regression included perinatal, neonatal, and biochemical variables. At term we found that the hours of oxygen (log) were a significant negative correlate of acuity. The older these babies were at the time of enrollment, the worse their acuity. Maternal gravida also correlated negatively with acuity. The only positive correlate of acuity at term was the red blood cell PE EPA at the time the infant was enrolled. When only supplemented infants were considered, hours of oxygen were again a negative correlate of acuity, and the red blood cell PE EPA at enrollment correlated positively. Among n–3 supplemented infants only, the number of hours of mechanical (log) ventilation was a negative correlate of acuity at term.

At two months of age (48 weeks), the red blood cell PE DHA at 38 weeks (term) correlated with acuity. Among unsupplemented infants, the red blood cell PE DHA at enrollment correlated with acuity. We did not expect such a relationship between DHA status and acuity among unsupplemented infants. However, DHA did fall to extremely low levels in some unsupplemented infants, and others maintain reasonably good levels of phospholipid DHA. Since our hypothesis was that DHA status would be a correlate of better acuity, these results are perhaps quite reasonable.

At four months of age, red blood cell PE DHA at enrollment was an important correlate of acuity. Formula with very long chain n–3 fatty acids was also. Among unsupplemented infants, no variables were significantly related to acuity at four months. Among n–3 supplemented infants, red blood cell PE EPA at 57 weeks correlated positively with acuity. I would emphasize here, therefore, that the individual DHA status of both unsupplemented and supplemented infants correlated with acuity.

Because the red blood cell PE DHA was so frequently a correlate of acuity, we asked yet another question: What factors are related to red blood cell PE DHA? At the time we enrolled these babies, the postnatal age at start was the major factor related to RBC PE DHA with older infants having lower DHA. Dr Innis showed you some data that are similar, showing that DHA decreases with time. We consistently see that the age of the baby at the time of enrollment is an important determinant of red blood cell DHA. This has nothing to do with gestational age because in general at whatever age these babies were born, their DHA status appears to be quite good. At term, consumption of n–3 supplemented formula only accounted for about 35% of the variance in RBC PE DHA, but by two and four months of age, n–3 supplementation accounted for about 80% of the variance in RBC PE DHA levels.

In summary, n–3 supplementation prevented declines in RBC PE DHA. Despite the inclusion of 3%–5% linolenic acid in both formulas, additional supplementation with very long chain n–3 fatty acids accounted for half of red blood cell phospholipid DHA after two months of age. N–3 supplemented infants had significantly improved acuity compared to controls. At term, acuity was inversely related to the hours of oxygen and ventilatory support, but these variables did not enter the regression model at later ages. Acuity at two and four months was positively related to the amount of DHA in red blood cell phospholipids, especially PE.

In conclusion, acuity was significantly improved in preterm infants by supplementation of linolenic acid-containing formulas with a marine oil source of very long chain n–3 fatty acids. Furthermore, n–3 fatty acid status was quite variable within each dietary group and predicted visual acuity regardless of dietary treatment. Other neonatal or perinatal variables also influenced acuity: hours of oxygen, mechanical ventilation, and maternal gravida. Membrane phospholipid DHA was influenced by postnatal age at enrollment and the infusion of very long chain n–3 fatty acids in formula.

Discussion

Chairman: Thank you very much for this very interesting communication. This is the first time that we have data on children having been fed with very long chain n–3 fatty acids in the diet.

S. Carlson: We are doing vitamin E and vitamin A analyses on these babies. These variables have not been included in this model since the analyses are incomplete. Vitamin E status seems to be all right although we do see some very low plasma vitamin A concentrations in the early term and two-month points. We do want to test whether this is related to acuity or cognition. Both vitamin E and vitamin A are known to affect photoreceptors in the retina.

J. Ghisolfi: Do you have any comment on the decrease of DHA concentration in brain, retina after you have stopped supplementation?

S. Carlson: These are data from living babies.

J. Ghisolfi: Yes, do you have any data about the monkeys?

S. Carlson: For the monkey data, I refer you to Neuringer and Connor's data. They have published data on fatty acid composition of both brain and retina. In some monkeys they have reversed the ERG abnormalities of n–3 deficiency by refeeding with fish oils. The data of Neuringer and Connor show that the brain is depleted of DHA. I just did not show you those slides today. I did, however, want to point out that these babies' plasma phospholipids are in the deficient range.

S. Innis: What effect does marine oil feeding have on n–6/n–3 ratio?

S. Carlson: I did not present that because that is published already in the *Federation Proceedings* from this year. We do see a decline in the n–6/n–3 ratio with marine oil feeding. As you saw, the EPA goes up. At the same time, arachidonic acid declines in plasma and red blood cell phospholipids. I cannot recall the n–6/n–3 ratio precisely, but I think it may decline by more than a half. You also asked about the type of formula fed. Infants receive preterm formula with about 20% linoleic acid, 3% linolenic, and medium chain triglycerides initially. They are changed to a term formula at approximately 1800 grams. The formula they go home on has about 35% linoleic and 5% linolenic acid; the ratio of n–6 to n–3 is about 7:1. Both term and preterm formulas contain 0.2% DHA and 0.3% EPA (g/100 g of total fatty acis).

M. Vidailhet: In your slides, mean ventilation was 66 hours in the protocol population. The mean was just 30 hours of ventilation in the supplemented population.

S. Carlson: You want me to explain that. That is very easy to explain. Some variables do not have a random distribution. Within both groups of infants there are babies who received no ventilatory support and others who received many hours. This is why the means do not differ and this variation can only be accounted for using a regression analysis.

C. Galli: I was very much interested in the relationship between DHA and EPA in the non-supplemented and supplemented babies. Is this the first observation showing the role of delta-4 desaturation activity?

S. Carlson: Well, as you know, there are no data on babies indicating their ability to desaturate at the delta-4 position. These data do suggest, however, that babies have a relative inability to form DHA at the rate they need DHA.

Chairman: Are there any pharmacological effects of feeding fish oil such as have been observed in the adult? Since you increase EPA in the red blood cells, have you looked at platelet aggregation?

S. Carlson: We have not looked at the platelets, but we looked at the superoxide production and do not see any difference between the production of superoxide by stimulated PMNs. I have been speaking with Dr Uauy's group in Dallas who are supplementing with twice as much marine oil as we. They find no significant effect on bleeding time. I really did not emphasize this enough, but we used a very low level of supplementation compared to the studies with adults that you may be aware of. On the other hand, we are feeding low levels of marine oil for a rather long period of time so, of course, we are looking for negative effects.

B. Koletzko: You chose to analyze red blood cells, and I wonder when you compare plasma and red blood cells in composition, do you draw the conclusion that the changes are relatively similar?

S. Carlson: Yes, they are similar when the infants are equilibrated on the diet for a number of months. For the most part, plasma DHA falls first, then red blood cell DHA falls later. Eventually they equilibrate. If you begin to supplement with DHA, the plasma DHA increases first and then red blood cell DHA increases later. I do feel that plasma PE analysis is more difficult technically than RBC PE, however.

Chairman: So one more question.

J. Rigo: Do you test the duration of total parenteral nutrition in the two groups?

S. Carlson: That is part of the analysis in the stepwise regression in the statistical analysis. The number of hours of total parenteral nutrition was the same in both groups. We tend to start our infants on enteral feeds between 48 and 72 hours of age.

J. Rigo: And did you test the taurine level of the baby?

S. Carlson: We have not measured taurine, but, of course, these babies are getting taurine.

J. Rigo: Is there any taurine in the formula?

S. Carlson: Yes, both the term and preterm formula are fortified with taurine.

D. Hull: Can I ask you about the normal values of visual acuity? What were these infants fed and were they premature?

S. Carlson: I would like to know the answer to that question also. It is relatively uncommon in the United States for babies to be breast fed to six months of age. I think it would be safe to say it is probably a group of term infants who have received human milk, formula, or a combination of human milk and formula during the first six months.

D. Hull: If you fed them human milk from the beginning, would you get this accelerated visual acuity?

S. Carlson: I do not know the answer to that question because we have not had a group of breast fed term infants to study. Those who developed these tests are not particularly interested in nutrition. They just wanted to know the visual acuity norms for babies. The norms were developed in the United States, and most American women do not breast feed beyond two months. Margit Hamosh may have some comments on this.

M. Hamosh: It depends; the higher socioeconomic strata have been better educated, and they will breast feed up to six months. The latest statistics on this came out about two weeks ago.

S. Carlson: I think the group probably had mixed feeding.

J. Rey: Do you think it is really an advantage to breast feed premature babies?

S. Carlson: Human milk possibly contributes uniquely to needs of the premature infant because it is a biological mixture similar to what the baby is getting *in utero*. Certain chemicals the baby would get *in utero* which are not in formula are in human milk; e.g., docosahexaenoic acid. However, there is ample evidence that preterm human milk is too low in calcium and phosphorus. The protein issue is still being debated by people who know far more about it than I do. So without question preterm human milk has certain nutrient deficiencies for the premature. Nevertheless, some compounds unique to human milk could be advantageous.

B. Salle: I think Rey was asking a very important question, but it is not only omega-3 fatty acid or polyunsaturated fatty acid. It is difficult to answer this question only on your data, but we have a lot of data about protein immunoglobulins, etc., into human milk.

S. Carlson: Yes, I think there are very many compounds in human milk that are not in formulas, and I would not be rash enough to say that preterm babies would not be at an advantage to get some of those compounds. We are just looking at one.

Chairman: So thank you very much.

12

Lipids in human milk and their digestion by the newborn infant

M. HAMOSH*, S.J. IVERSON*, N.R. MEHTA*, M.L. SPEAR**, J. BITMAN***

* *Department of Pediatrics, Georgetown University Children's Medical Center, 3800 Reservoir Road NW, Washington, DC 20007-2197, USA.*
** *Division of Neonatology, Medical Center of Delaware and E. Jefferson Medical College, Philadelphia, PA, USA.*
*** *Milk Secretion and Mastitis Laboratory, USDA-ARS, Beltsville, MD, USA.*

Accretion of essential fatty acids occurs usually during the last trimester of pregnancy. Several presentations at this workshop have addressed the aspects of *in utero* supply of fatty acids to the foetus and the role of the placenta in this process.

In this chapter, we would like to concentrate on two main topics that address the postnatal supply of essential fatty acids to the newborn infant, namely the composition of milk lipids and their digestion by the infant. After birth, the source of essential fatty acids is human milk or infant formula. However, infant formulas do not contain long chain polyunsaturated fatty acids containing greater than 18 carbon atoms. Furthermore, the ability of the infant to utilize these fatty acids will depend upon their efficient release during the digestive process. Because of differences in the composition of the lipids in milk produced by mothers who deliver preterm as compared to full term infants, we will briefly address this topic.

Composition of human milk

Fat is the most variable component of human milk, changing as a function of length of gestation, length of lactation, time of day, duration of individual feeds (low in fore and high in hind milk) as well as maternal diet [1]. Because of insolubility in aqueous media, the fat in milk is contained in specific structures, the milk fat globules. These consist of a triglyceride core and a membrane composed mainly of polar lipids (phospholipids and cholesterol) and proteins. The changes in milk fat content and composition are most pronounced during early lactation and during weaning. The type and amount of dietary fat affect the composition of milk to a great extent. Thus, maternal diets low in fat and high in carbohydrate lead to *de novo* synthesis of fatty acids within the mammary gland, resulting in high concentrations of fatty acids of chain length ≤ C16. Therefore, although the total amount of fat will remain in the normal range, milk fat will be much more saturated, because these fatty acids (C8-C16) are all saturated. Shifts in dietary practices of populations result in changes in the fatty acid composition of human milk. For example, in the United States the increased consumption of vegetable oils has led to an increase of linoleic acid in human milk from approximately 8% in the 1960-1970's to 15% in the 1980's [1, 2]. A similar increase in long chain polyunsaturated fatty acids, such as docosahexaenoic acid (C22:ω6), in human milk in the USA can be expected as a result of the increased consumption of fish, rich in these fatty acids.

The first tables and figures provide data on the fat composition of human milk as well as on the effects of length of gestation and lactation on milk fat.

Mature milk (i.e. after completion of the transition from colostrum) has a fat content of 3.5-4.5% *(Table I)*. There are, however, individual variations indicating that some women produce constantly milk with high or low fat throughout lactation. Infant growth is not affected, because production of milk with low fat concentration is associated with the secretion of higher volumes of milk [3].

Table I. Composition of human milk fat[*]

Glycerides		3.0-4.5 mg/dl	
Triglycerides	98.70%+		Major component
Diglycerides	0.01%		of the core of
Monoglycerides	0		milk fat globules
Free Fatty Acids	0.08%		
Cholesterol		10-15 mg/dl	
			Major component of milk fat globule
Phospholipids		15-20 mg/dl	membrane
Sphingomyelin	37%		
Phosphatidylcholine	28%		
Phosphatidylserine	9%		
Phosphatidylinositol	6%		
Phosphatidylethanolamine	19%		

Data from Hamosh M., Bitman J., Wood D.L., *et al.* Lipids in milk and the first steps in their digestion. *Pediatrics* 1985; 75 (Suppl): 146-50. [*]Mature milk from mothers of term infants. + Percent in lipid class (glycerides and phopholipids, respectively).

The main component of human milk fat are the triglycerides (98-99% of total fat), whereas phospholipids and cholesterol are present at much lower levels (15-20 mg/dl and 10-15 mg/dl, respectively). As mentioned above, the triglycerides are located in the core of milk fat globules, whereas the polar lipids (phospholipids and cholesterol) form the membrane of the milk fat globules.

Whereas the amount of triglyceride remains constant throughout lactation, the concentration of phospholipids and cholesterol decreases markedly during the first 3 weeks of lactation (*figures 1A and 1B*). This decrease is even more drastic in preterm milk because of the higher levels of phospholipid and cholesterol in colostrum. The decline in phospholipid and cholesterol levels agrees well with an increase in the fat globule size [5, 6], and thus a decrease in the amount of membrane lipids.

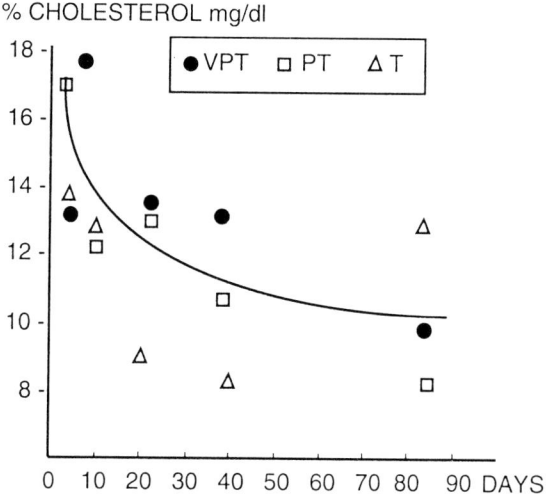

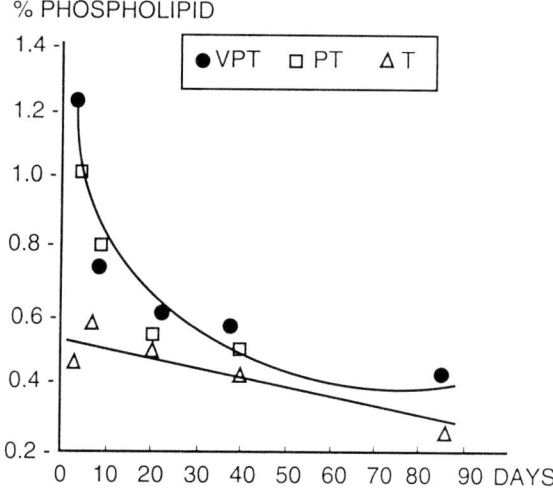

Figure 1. Changes in the concentration of cholesterol and phospholipid in milk of mothers of preterm and fullterm infants during lactation. Milk was from mothers delivering at 26-30 wks (VPT), 31-36 wks. (PT) and 37-40 wks (T) gestation.
A. Cholesterol. (Data from Bitman *et al. Am J Clin Nutr* 1983; 38:300-12).
B. Phospholipid. (Data from Bitman *et al. Am J Clin Nutr* 1984; 40: 1103-19).

The fatty acid composition of milk secreted by American women (mothers of premature and full term infants) is shown in *Table II*. The data are representative of a total of 52 women (18 in the VPT-very premature group, gestational age 26-30 weeks; 28 in the PT group-premature, gestational age 31-36 weeks; and 6 in term-T group, gestational age 37-40 weeks. Milk was collected on day 42 of lactation, thus representing mature milk. *Table II* shows that over 98% of the fat in human milk is present in 11 major fatty acids from C10:0 to C20:4. Differences are seen in certain milk fatty acid levels among the three groups of women: medium chain fatty acids ≤ C14 amount to 10% of total fatty acids in milk of mothers of full term infants, but contribute 17% of total fatty acids in milk produced by mothers of preterm infants. Furthermore, essential fatty acid contents are higher in colostrum and transitional milk than in mature milk. Long chain polyunsaturated fatty acids derived from linoleic acid (ω6), 20:2, 20:3, 20:4 and 22:5, and from linolenic acid (ω3), 20:5, 22:5, 22:6, show a similar decrease throughout lactation. The level of these fatty acids is significantly higher in colostrum and milk of mothers of preterm infants than of mothers of full term infants (*figure 2*). Thus, preterm infants fed their

Table II. Milk lipids of mothers of preterm and full term infants

Fatty acid composition of human milk fat at day 42 of lactation: comparison of milk from mothers who delivered at 26 to 30 wk (VPT), 31 to 36 wk (PT), and 37 to 40 wk (T) of pregnancy

Fatty acid	VPT* 26-30 wk	PT 31-36 wk	T 37-40 wk
10:0	1.37 ± 0.17	1.27 ± 0.18	0.97 ± 0.28
12:0	7.47 ± 0.72	6.55 ± 0.77	4.46 ± 1.17
14:0	8.41 ± 0.83	7.55 ± 0.89	5.68 ± 1.36
15:0	0.23 ± 0.04	0.27 ± 0.05	0.31 ± 0.07
16:0	20.13 ± 1.40	23.16 ± 1.49	22.20 ± 2.28
16:1	2.56 ± 0.24	2.92 ± 0.26	3.83 ± 0.39
17:0	0.34 ± 0.22	0.60 ± 0.24	0.49 ± 0.36
18:0	7.24 ± 1.13	7.25 ± 1.21	7.68 ± 1.85
18:1	33.41 ± 1.67	33.74 ± 1.79	35.51 ± 2.73
18:2	15.75 ± 1.22	13.83 ± 1.30	15.58 ± 1.99
18:3	0.76 ± 0.13	0.76 ± 0.14	1.03 ± 0.21
20:0	0.17 ± 0.07	0.09 ± 0.14	0.32 ± 0.11
20:2	0.35 ± 0.13	0.33 ± 0.13	0.18 ± 0.20
20:3	0.51 ± 0.09	0.43 ± 0.10	0.53 ± 0.15
20:4	0.55 ± 0.18	0.58 ± 0.19	0.60 ± 0.29
20:5	0.04 ± 0.05	0.00	0.00
21:0	0.05 ± 0.07	0.07 ± 0.08	0.07 ± 0.16
22:4	0.13 ± 0.10	0.24 ± 0.11	0.03 ± 0.08
22:5ω6	0.11 ± 0.05	0.04 ± 0.05	0.03 ± 0.08
22:5ω3	0.42 ± 0.09	0.12 ± 0.12	0.11 ± 0.15
22:6	0.24 ± 0.09	0.21 ± 0.09	0.23 ± 0.14

* Means ± SE.
Data are from Bitman *et al. Am J Clin Nutr* 1983; 38; 300-13.

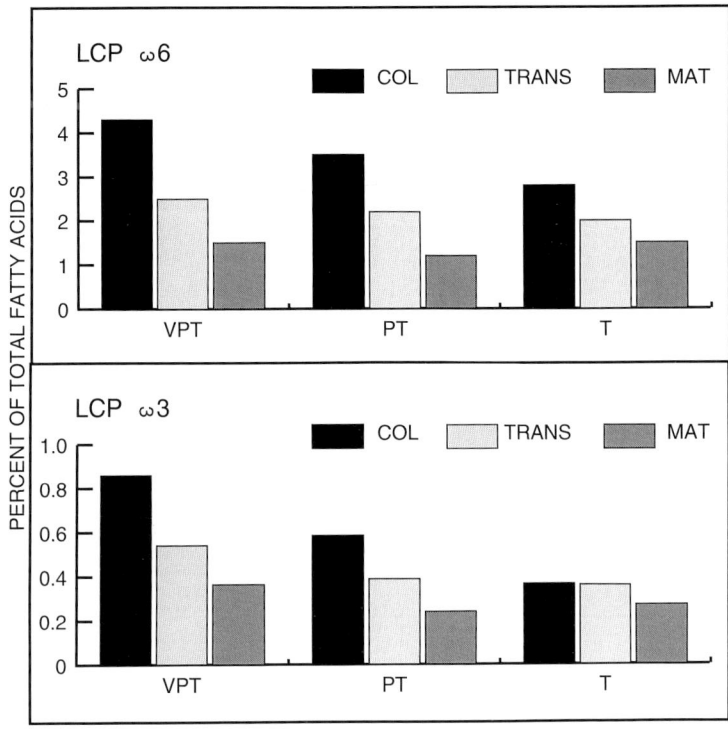

Figure 2. Concentrations of long chain polyunsaturated fatty acids (C20 and C22) in human milk fat derived from either linoleic (LCP-W6) or linolenic acid (LCP-W3). Milk was from mothers of infants of gestational age 26-30 wks (VPT), 31-36 wks (PT) and 37-40 wks (T). COL: colostrum (3 days post partum); TRANS: transitional milk (7 days post partum); MAT: mature milk (21 days post partum). (Data from Bitman *et al. Am J Clin Nutr* 1983; 38:300-12).

mother's milk receive adequate amounts of long chain polyunsaturated fatty acids required for neural tissue synthesis [7].

Milk phospholipids and cholesterol esters contain higher concentrations of essential unsaturated and polyunsaturated fatty acids than do triglycerides (*Table III* and *figure 3*). Within the phospholipid classes there is a slight but definite increase in the unsaturated nature of the glycerides, the degree of unsaturation increasing in the order of PE > PI > PS > PC. Sphingomyelin is the largest phospholipid class and is also the most saturated (80% saturated fatty acids, as compared to 40 and 50% in the other phospholipids). Furthermore, sphingomyelin contains a large percentage of fatty acids > C22 (C23-6.2 to 7.7%, C24:0 – 15.6 to 17.9% and C24:1 – 9.7 to 17.7%). As can be seen from *figure 3*, 73% of the fatty acids in cholesteryl esters are unsaturated as compared to 52% unsaturated fatty acids in triglycerides [8].

Fatty acids of chain length in excess of C18 are produced by elongation and desaturation of the precursor linoleic (C18:2ω6) and linolenic (C18:3ω3) acids. These long chain polyunsaturated fatty acids (> C18) can also be provided by the diet, if

Table III. Essential fatty acids in the phospholipids of human milk

Fatty Acid (wt %)	Phospholipid Classes[*]				Total Fat[**] (wt %)
	PE	PI	PS	PC	
18:2	20.8	19.5	23.0	21.0	15.5
18:3	2.9	1.7	2.0	0.8	1.0
20:2	0.9	0.8	0.4	0.3	0.2
20:3	2.2	4.4	3.0	1.1	0.5
20:4	8.4	7.0	3.4	2.4	0.6
20:5	0	–	0	0	0
22:4	2.2	1.8	2.2	0.5	0.07
22:5ω6	1.7	1.6	1.9	0.4	0.03
22:5ω3	0.9	0.5	0.7	0.1	0.1
22:6ω3	1.6	1.3	1.5	0.3	0.2

[*] PE: phosphatidylethanolamine, PI: phosphatidylinositol, PS: phosphatidylserine, PC: phosphatidylcholine.
[**] Total milk fat.
The data are for mature milk (days 21-84 post partum) of mothers of full term infants. From Bitman et al. Am J Clin Nutr 1984; 40: 1103-1119.

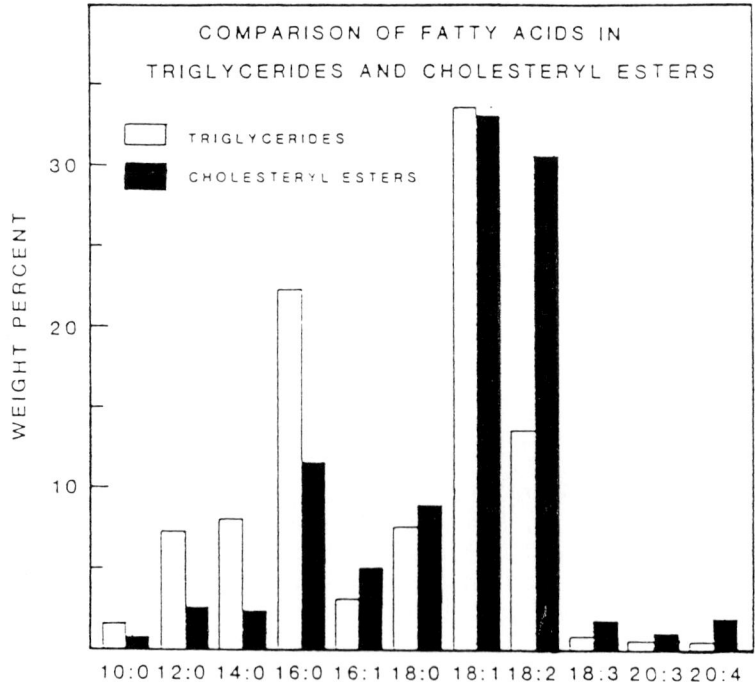

Figure 3. Comparison of fatty acids in triglycerides and cholesterol esters of mature human milk. (Data from Bitman et al. J Pediatr Gastroenterol Nutr 1986; 5: 780-6).

the latter is rich in fish or fish oil. In order to assess the ability of the lactating mammary gland to produce these fatty acids we have used the milk to plasma ratio as an indicator of fatty acid origin, i.e. a ratio close to 1 indicates uptake from the circulation, thus dietary or fat depot origin, while a ratio > 1 would indicate production within the mammary gland. The data presented, based on the analysis of colostrum and plasma lipids of 30 mothers of full term infants studied within the first two days after parturition, show that there is extensive elongation and desaturation in the mammary gland shortly after parturition. Furthermore, the higher concentration of long chain polyunsaturated fatty acids in colostrum of women who deliver prematurely (*figure 4*) indicates that elongation and desaturation capacity is present in the mammary gland immediately after parturition and is independent of duration of pregnancy.

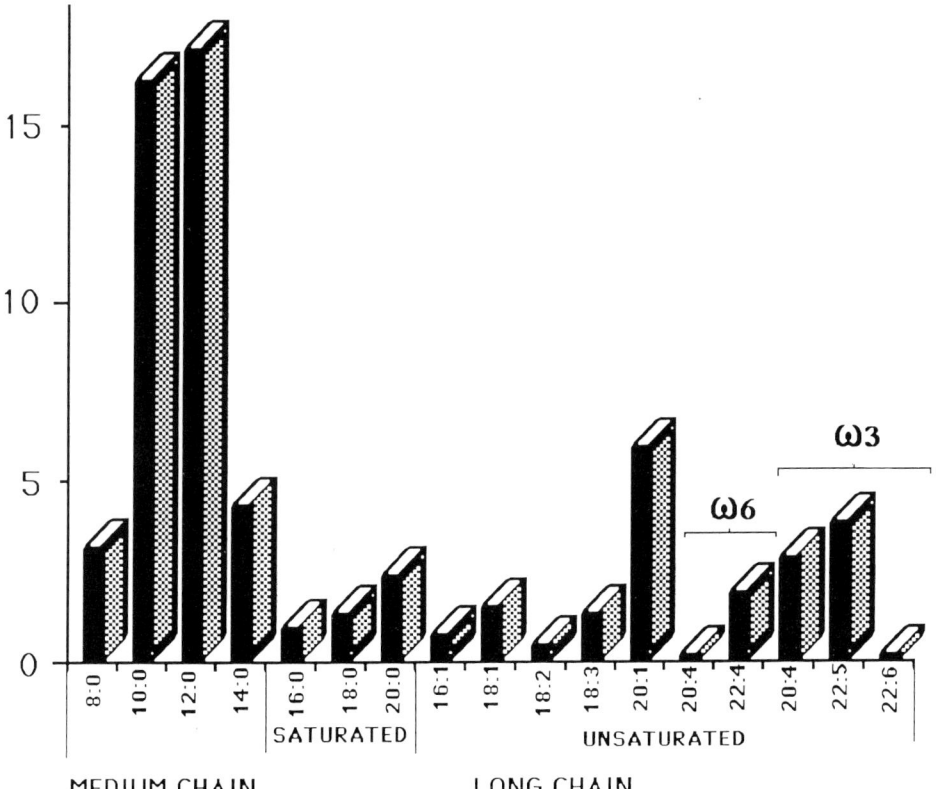

Figure 4. Fatty acid elongation and desaturation in the lactating mammary gland. Milk: plasma fatty acid ratios. Plasma and milk fatty acids were analyzed by GLC. Ratios in excess of 1:0 indicate production within the mammary gland. (Data from Hamosh *et al.*, in press, 1990).

Digestion of milk fat

In order for the individual essential fatty acids to be metabolized by the various organs of the body, milk fat has first to be digested and absorbed. Digestion of fat is initiated in the stomach through the action of lingual and gastric lipases [10]. These enzymes (the first secreted from the lingual serous glands and the second from the gastric mucosa) have an amino acid homology close to 80% and very similar characteristics (Table IV). This first step in fat digestion is then continued in the duodenum by pancreatic lipase and the milk's own digestive lipase (which has characteristics close to those of pancreatic lipase, i.e. an absolute requirement for bile salt concentrations > CMC and a pH optimum > 6.0-6.5 [11]). Initial fat hydrolysis in the stomach is necessary for optimal fat digestion and absorption at all ages [12, 13]. This step is, however, of significantly greater importance in the newborn because of endogenous and exogenous reasons. The first is low pancreatic lipase activity in the newborn and especially the preterm infant [14], while the second refers to the nature of the lipid digested, milk fat globules being inaccessible to both pancreatic lipase [12, 15] as well as milk digestive lipase [16]. Indeed as shown in *figure 5A,* initial digestion of milk fat by lingual lipase is essential for the subsequent hydrolysis of milk fat by pancreatic lipase [16], while as seen in *figure 5B,* the fat in either human milk or infant formula is inaccessible to the milk digestive lipase, resulting in only minimal lipolysis, unless both types of lipid were first digested by lingual lipase [16]. Indeed, not only does partial digestion by lingual lipase facilitate the subsequent digestion by milk lipase, in addition it enables the latter to hyodrolyze lipid even in the absence of bile salts (*figure 5*). The specific characteristics of lingual and gastric lipase (hydrophobicity, inability to hydrolyze the ester bonds of phospholipids and cholesteryl esters as well as stimulation of activity by dietary proteins that reduce interfacial pressure to the range optimal for these enzymes) indicate that these enzymes are ideally suited to initiate the digestion of fat in milk fat globules, by being able to penetrate through the milk fat globule membrane without disrupting it (*figure 6*) [17, 18].

Table IV. Characteristics and requirements for optimal activity of digestive lipases

Condition	Lingual	Gastric	Pancreatic	Milk
TG-site (Sn)	Sn 3	Sn 3	Sn 1, 3	Sn 1, 2, 3
Pred ct	1,2 DG (MG)	1,2 DG (MG)	2 MG	FFA
pH Optimum	2.2-6.0	3.5-6.5	6.5-8.0	7.0-8.5
Cofactors	none	none	colipase	none
Bile salts	no	no	> CMC	> CMC
Stability (pH 2.5-3.0)	yes	yes	no	yes
Protein	stimulation	stimulation	inhibition	no effect

TG – triglyceride; Sn – stereospecific numbering
DG – diglyceride; MG – monoglyceride

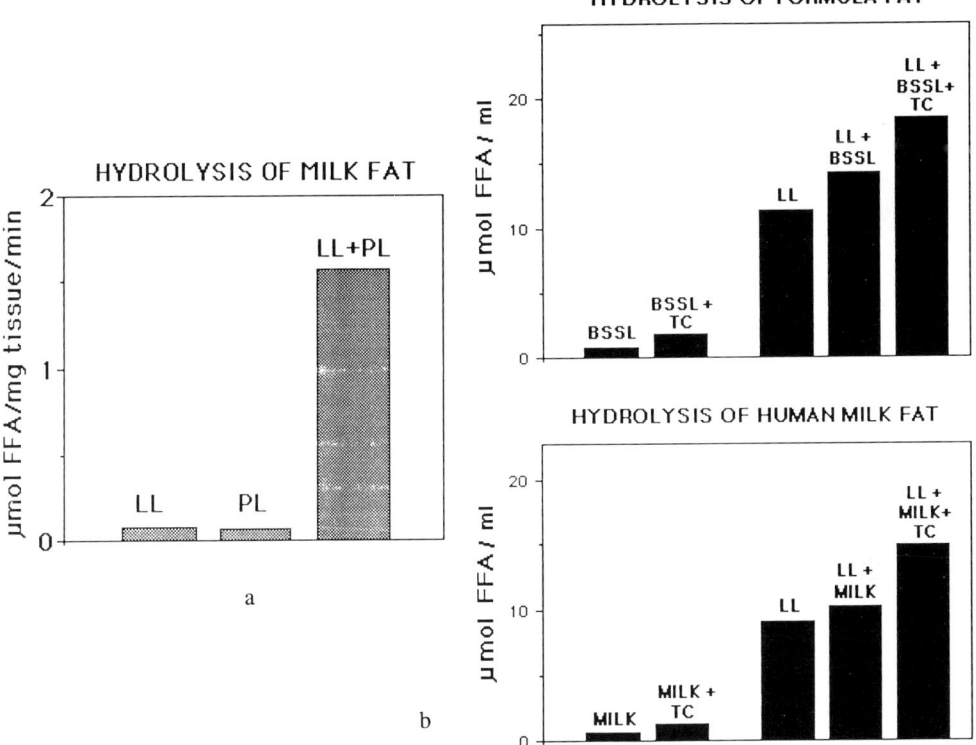

Figure 5. Facilitating role of initial digestion by lingual lipase on the subsequent lipolysis of milk fat by pancreatic lipase and milk digestive lipase.
A. Pancreatic lipase: Lingual lipase (LL), incubation 30 min, pH 5.4; pancreatic lipase (PL) incubation 30 min, pH 8.0, 4mM sodium taurocholate; LL + PL: lingual lipase incubation, 30 min, pH 5.4 followed by change of pH to 8.0, addition of 4mM sodium taurocholate and pancreatic lipase. Substrate milk fat. Lipolytic activity: μmol FFA released/min/mg tissue. Preincubation of milk fat with lingual lipase leads to a 20 fold enhancement of the activity of pancreatic lipase. (From Plucinski et al. Am J Physiol 1979; 237:E541-E547). **B. Milk digestive lipase**: BSSL – milk bile salt stimulated lipase, TC – taurocholate: columns 1 and 2 minimal hydrolysis of dietary fat during 1 hour incubation, LL – lingual lipase: incubation for 1 h with LL leads to marked hydrolysis of fat and enhances the subsequent action of BSSL (columns 3-5) Upper panel: Substrate formula fat, BSSL – fresh human skim milk. Lower panel: fresh human milk provided both substrate and BSSL activity. (From Hamosh M., Development of Lipid metabolism. In: Xanthou, ed. *New aspects of nutrition in infancy and prematurity.* Amsterdam: Elsevier; 1987: 67-78).

Although it was generally assumed that during the gastric phase of fat digestion, the fatty acids released are mainly short and medium chain fatty acids [15], more recent studies show that long chain unsaturated fatty acids are also preferentially hydrolyzed [17, 19, 20]. In *in vitro* studies, conducted under conditions simulating the gastric milieu *in vivo* [17], it is clearly evident that long chain unsaturated fatty

Essential fatty acids and infant nutrition

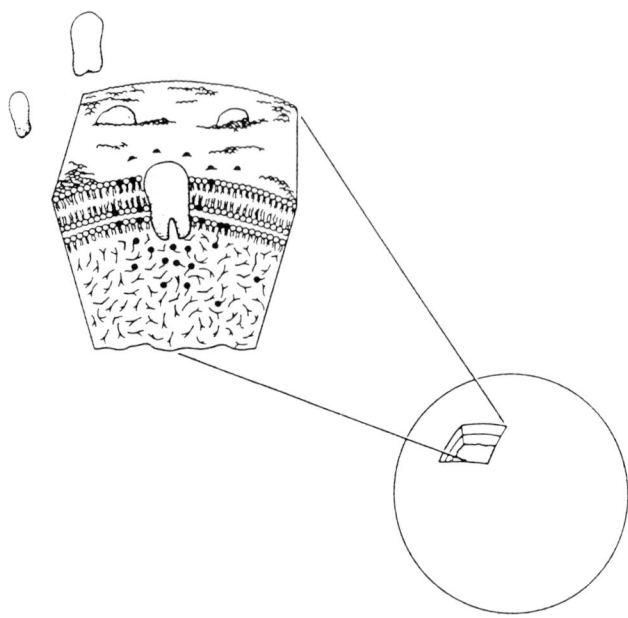

Figure 6. Hydrolysis of milk fat globule triglyceride by lingual lipase. Schematic drawing based on data that show that although as much as 15% of triglyceride is hydrolyzed to FFA and partial glycerides, there is no change in the appearance of the milk fat globules (Patton J.S., *et al. Biochim Biophys Acta* 1982; 712:400-7). Enzyme molecules penetrate the membrane of the globule and hydrolyze the triglycerides in the core fat (shown as forked sticks) to fatty acids (black tipped sticks) and diglycerides (darkened sticks) which remain associated with the droplet (From Hamosh M. Lingual Lipase. In: Borgstrom B., Brockman H.L., eds. *Lipases*. Amsterdam: Elsevier, 1984; 49-84.

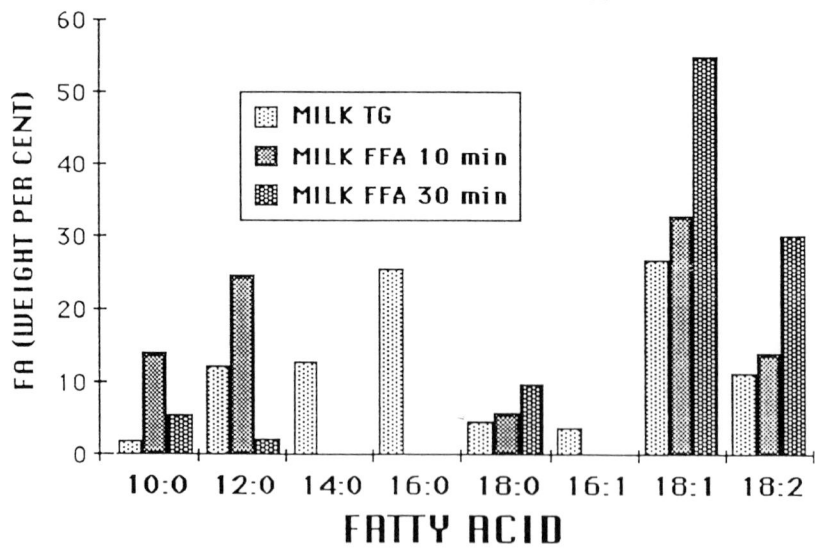

Figure 7. Hydrolysis of human milk fat by lingual lipase: *in vitro* studies. (Incubation at pH 5.4.) (Data from Patton *et al. Biochim Biophys Acta* 1982; 712: 400-7).

acids (i.e. oleic and linoleic) are preferentially released from human milk fat by lingual lipase (*figure 7*). The study shows that medium chain fatty acids (C12-C14) are also readily released from milk fat, while longer chain saturated fatty acids (C14:0 and C16:0) are not cleaved from the triglyceride molecule. This specificity could be associated not only with the nature of the fatty acid, but also with the position of the fatty acid in the triglyceride molecule; for example palmitic acid, C16:0, is located at position Sn2, which is not hydrolyzed by many digestive lipases, such as lingual and pancreatic lipases. Likewise, the composition of the free fatty acids produced during gastric lipolysis in one day old suckling rat pups shows preferential release of medium chain (C8:0-C14:0) and long chain unsaturated (C18:1-C18:3) fatty acids [19] (*figure 8*). Furthermore, the greatest increment of individual fatty acids released was in the long chain polyunsaturated ones (C20:3). Thus, while saturated long chain fatty acids (C16:0-C18:0) are not hydrolyzed (resulting in a proportional enrichment of the milk triglycerides in these fatty acids), long chain unsaturated and polyunsaturated fatty acids (i.e. essential fatty acids) are readily released during gastric lipolysis in the rat. Fat digestion differs, however, greatly between the rat and the human. Rat milk does not contain a digestive lipase, whereas the only endogenous preduodenal lipase is lingual lipase [10]. The human has both lingual and gastric lipases [21, 22], whereas the milk contains also a diges-

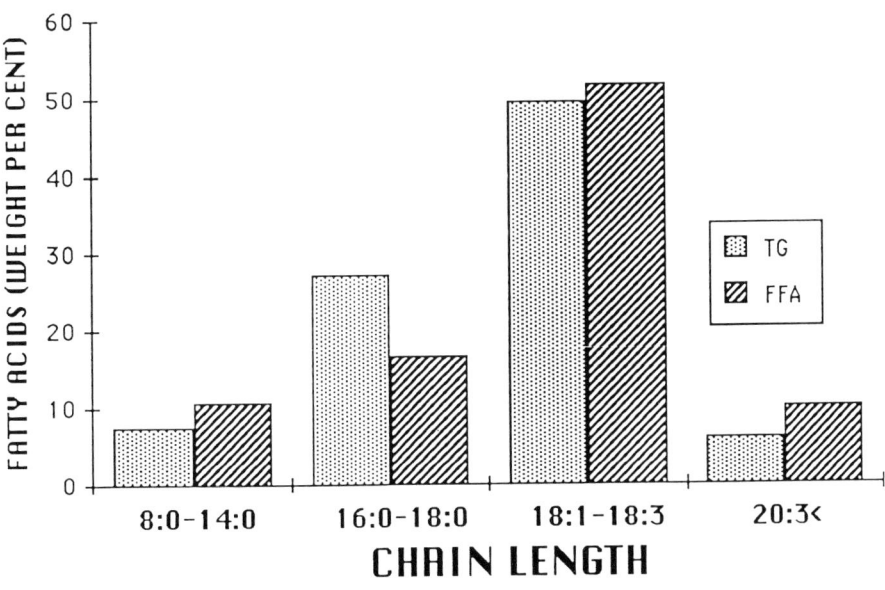

Figure 8. Hydrolysis of rat milk in the stomach of 1 day old pups. *In vivo* studies. Gastric contents taken 30 min after milk feeding. (Data from Bitman *et al. Biochim Biophys Acta* 1985; 834:58-64).

tive lipase. The dog, a species with gastric lipase and milk digestive lipase, identical to that of the human, seems an ideal model to study digestion of milk fat in the newborn. Thus, studies in the dog permit a quantitative assessment of the extent of *in vivo* lipolysis and comparison with *in vitro* conditions that simulate the gastric milieu. This type of comparison is important, since most of our knowledge in this field is based on *in vitro* studies that have used gastric or lingual lipase and either artificial lipid emulsions or fresh milk as substrate. We have recently carried out such studies in the dog [24]. These studies (*figure 9*) show that *in vitro* experiments, using fresh dog milk fat as substrate and either pinch biopsy specimens of gastric mucosa from suckling dog puppies as source of gastric lipase, or the fresh milk's own digestive lipase, greatly underestimate the digestive potential of the stomach. Thus, while *in vitro*, under optimal assay conditions (pH 5) and fatty acid acceptor for gastric lipase, and pH 8.5 and bile salts for the milk digestive lipase, gastric lipase hydrolyzed only 13% of milk fat while the milk lipase was able to

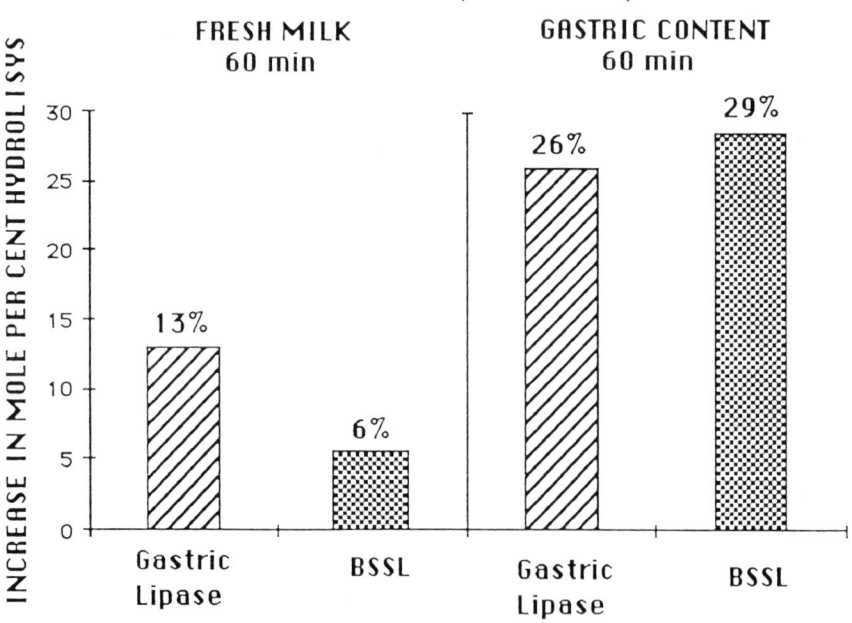

Figure 9. *In vitro* hydrolysis of milk fat in the puppy dog after and prior to intragastric lipolysis. At 4 wks post partum, freshly collected milk was incubated with gastric mucosa biopsies from puppies in assay systems specific for gastric and milk lipase activity (i.e. pH 5.1 and BSA or pH 8.5, BSA and bile salts, respectively). Left Panel. Gastric aspirates from the same puppies were concurrently incubated in the same systems for comparison-right panel. Left panel-*in vitro* incubation 60 min. Right panel–*in vivo* 30 min after gavage feeding followed by 30 min *in vitro* incubation.

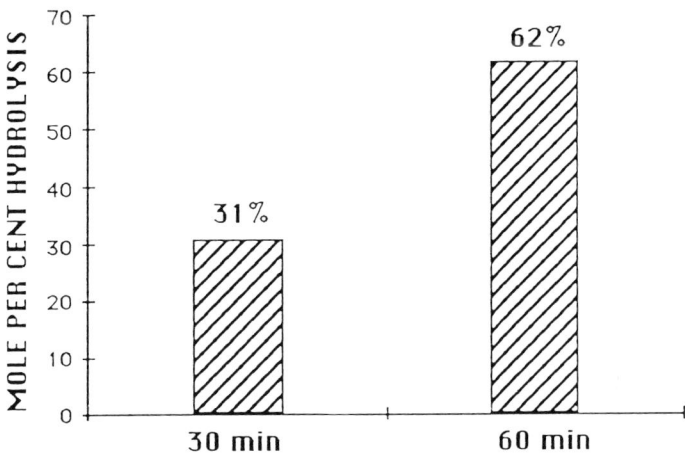

Figure 10. *In vitro* gastric hydrolysis of milk fat in the puppy.

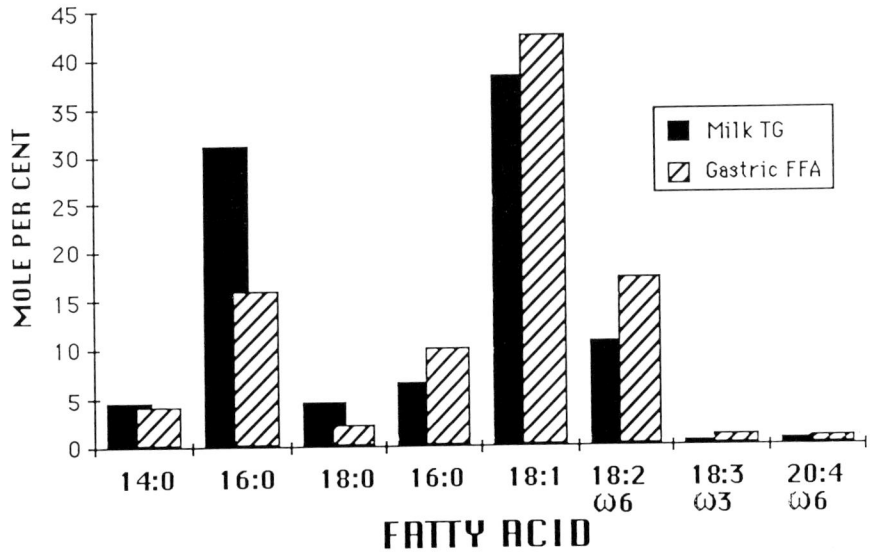

Figure 11. Hydrolysis of milk fat in the puppy. Comparison of fatty acid composition in the fatty acid and triglyceride fractions of gastric contents after gavage feeding of fresh dog milk.

hydrolyze only 6% of milk fat during one hour's incubation. However, when gastric contents were aspirated 30 min after gavage feeding and incubated for an additional 30 min *in vitro,* gastric lipase hydrolyzed 26% of milk fat, while milk lipase activity resulted in the hydrolysis of as much as 29% of milk fat. Thus, as previously shown in *in vitro* studies, partial lipolysis by gastric lipase is essential for the hydrolysis of milk fat by the milk digestive lipase.

Furthermore, quantitation of gastric lipolysis in 4 week old pups shows that as much as 62% of milk fat is hydrolyzed with one hour after milk ingestion (*figure 10*). Therefore, *in vivo,* gastric lipolysis of milk fat is not subject to the strong product inhibition described previously for both lingual [18] or gastric lipase [10] in *in vitro* studies with artificial fat emulsions. Examination of the composition of dog milk shows that it contains fatty acids of chain length of 14 to 20 carbons, thus mainly long chain fatty acids (*figure 11*). During gastric lipolysis essential fatty acids are preferentially released (*figure 10*). This study in the dog shows that milk fat containing mainly long chain fatty acids is rapidly and extensively hydrolyzed in the stomach of the newborn.

The ability of the newborn infant to release long chain fatty acids during intragastric lipolysis was recently examined [20]. This study shows that 15 min after gavage feeding preterm infant formula containing long chain triglycerides, the free

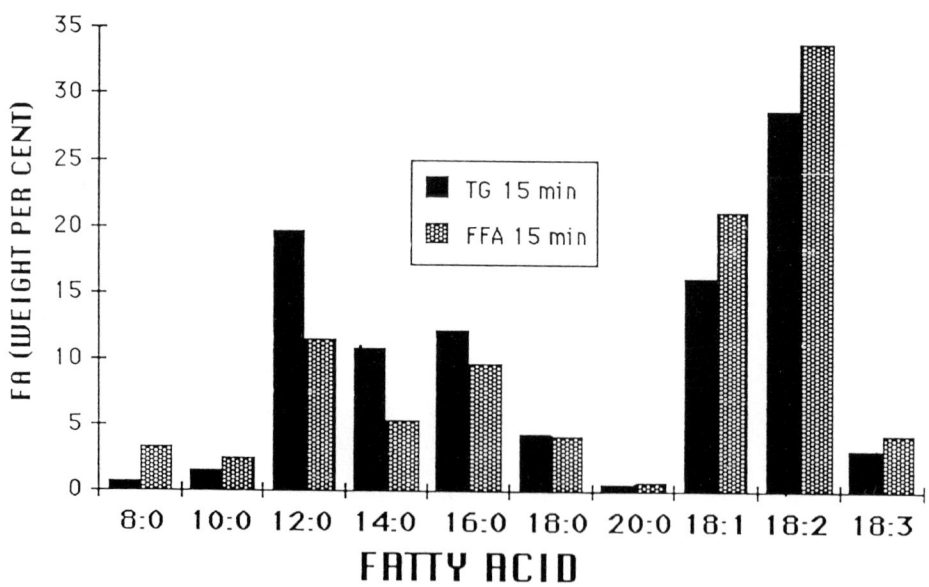

Figure 12. Hydrolysis of long chain triglyceride formula in the stomach of premature infants. Gastric contents were aspirated for fatty acid analysis, 15 min after gavage feeding. (Data from Hamosh *et al. Pediatrics* 1989; 83:86-92).

fatty acids in the stomach were enriched in medium and long chain unsaturated fatty acids, whereas the triglycerides were enriched in saturated fatty acids (*figure 12*). Thus, in the human infant, the process of gastric lipolysis also preferentially releases essential fatty acids in addition to medium chain fatty acids.

In conclusion: our studies show that long chain polyunsaturated fatty acids are synthesized in the mammary gland immediately after parturition and that the capacity of the human mammary gland to elongate and desaturate fatty acids is independent of length of gestation. Long chain polyunsaturated fatty acid concentrations are higher: *a* in colostrum than in mature milk, *b* in milk of women who deliver preterm and *c* in phospholipids and cholesterol esters than in triglycerides of human milk. Gastric digestion of milk fat can account for hydrolysis of 60% of the ingested fat and releases preferentially long chain mono and polyunsaturated fatty acids as well as medium chain fatty acids. This step is essential for the subsequent action of both milk digestive lipase as well as pancreatic lipase. *In vitro* studies that simulate the gastric milieu strongly underestimate the extent of gastric lipolysis.

Acknowledgement

The skillful secretarial help of Mrs. Dianne P. Jefferson is gratefully acknowledged. The authors' studies are supported by NIH grants HD-10823 and HD-20833 and by grants from Wyeth Ayerst Laboratories and the Mead Johnson Nutrition Division.

References

1. Jensen R.G. (1989) The lipids of human milk, Boca Raton: CRC Press, FL.
2. Bitman J., Wood D.L., Hamosh M., Hamosh P., Mehta N.R. (1983) Comparison of the lipid composition of breast milk from mothers of term and preterm infants. *Am J Clin Nutr* 38: 300-13.
3. Hachey D.L., Motil K.J., Wong W.W., Garza C., Klein P.D. (1989) Milk production and fat concentration are related to whole body water flux during human lactation. *FASEB J* 3: A454.
4. Bitman J., Wood D.L., Mehta N.R., Hamosh P., Hamosh M. (1984) Comparison of the phospholipid composition of breast milk from mothers of term and preterm infants during lactation. *Am J Clin Nutr* 40: 1103-19.
5. Ruegg M., Blanc B. (1981) The fat globule size distribution in human milk. *Biochim Biophys Acta* 666:7-12.
6. Simonin C., Ruegg M., Sidiropoulos D. (1984) Comparison of the fat content and fat globule size distribution of breast milk from mothers delivering term and preterm. *Am J Clin Nutr* 40: 820-5.
7. Clandinin M.T., Chappell J.E., Hern T. (1982) Do low weight infants require nutrition with chain elongation desaturation products of essential fatty acids? In: Holman R.T., ed. *Essential Fatty Acids and Prostaglandins.* New York: Pergamon Press, 901-15.
8. Bitman J., Wood D.L., Mehta N.R., Hamosh P., Hamosh M. (1982) Comparison of the cholesteryl ester composition of breast milk from preterm and term mothers *J Pediatr Gastroenterol Nutr* 6:780-6.

9. Harris W.S., Connor W.E., Lindsey S. (1984) Will dietary W3 fatty acids change the composition of human milk? *Am J Clin Nutr* 40:780-4.
10. Hamosh M., Hamosh P. (1989) Lingual and gastric lipases during development. In: Lebenthal E., ed. *Human Gastrointestinal Development.* New York: Raven Press, 251-76.
11. Hamosh M. (1988) Fat needs for term and preterm infants. In: Tsany R.C., Nichols B.L., eds. *Nutrition During Infancy.* St. Louis: CV Mosby Co, 133-59.
12. Plucinski T.M., Hamosh M. Hamosh P. (1979) Fat digestion in the rat: role of lingual lipase. *Am J Physiol* 237: E541-7.
13. Roy C.C., Roulet M., Leferbre D., Chartrand L., Lepage C., Fournier LA. (1979) The role of gastric lipolysis in fat absorption and bile acid metabolism in the rat. *Lipids* 14: 811-4.
14. Watkins J.B. (1975) Mechanism of fat absorption and the development of gastrointestinal function. *Pediatr Clin N Am* 22: 721-30.
15. Cohen M., Morgan G.R.H., Hofmann A.F. (1971) Lipolytic activity of human gastric and duodenal juice against medium and long-chain triglycerides. *Gastroenterology* 60: 1-15.
16. Hamosh M. (1988) Development of lipid metabolism. In: Xanthou M., ed. New aspects of nutrition in infancy and prematurity. Amsterdam: Elsevier, 67-78.
17. Patton J.S., Rigler M.W., Liao T.H., Hamosh P., Hamosh M. (1982) Hydrolysis of triacylglycerol emulsions by lingual lipase – a microscopic study. *Biochim Biophys Acta* 712:400-7.
18. Hamosh M. (1983) Lingual lipase. In: Borgstrom B., Brockman HL., eds. *Lipases.* Amsterdam: Elsevier, 49-82.
19. Bitman J., Wood D.L., Liao T.H., Fink C.S., Hamosh P., Hamosh M. (1985) Gastric lipolysis of milk lipids in suckling rats. *Biochim Biophys Acta* 834: 58-64.
20. Hamosh M., Bitman J., Liao T.H., Mehta N.R., Buczek R.J., Wood D.L., Grylack L.J., Hamosh P. (1989) Gastric lipolysis and fat absorption in preterm infants: effect of MCT or LCT containing formulas. *Pediatrics* 83:86-92.
21. Hamosh M., Burns W. (1977) Lipolytic activity of human lingual glands (Ebner). *Lab Invest* 37:603-8.
22. Salzman-Mann C., Hamosh M., Sivasubramanian K.N., et al. (1982) Congenital esophageal atresia: lipase activity is present in the esophageal pouch and in the stomach. *Dig Dis Sci* 27-124-8.
23. Hamosh M. (1988) Enzymes in milk: their function in the mammary gland, in milk and in the infant. In: Hanson L.A., ed. *Biology of Human Milk.* New York: Raven Press, 45-58.
24. Iverson J.J., Kirk C.L., Hamosh M. (1990) Fat digestion in the newborn: *in vitro* studies greatly underestimate the high extent of intragastric digestion of fat. *Pediatr Res* 27:107A.

Discussion

Chairman: So thank you very much for these very interesting indications. Do you have any questions?

G. Béréziat: In the first part of your talk, you said that in the mammary gland there is some synthesis of unsaturated fatty acids. Have you any evidence that in this tissue there is delta-5 or delta-6-desaturase activity.

M. Hamosh: No, we have not measured it; simply because we have worked with human milk and we have a very hard time getting biopsis from a lactating mother; as a matter of fact we wouldn't even try it. However your question will be answered in the very near future, because we are going now to use the dog and we are going to look at that; however the dog is limited as far as the long chain polyunsaturated are concerned, so we might have to go to another species which we are now looking at.

O. Hernell: I have a couple of questions, first it has been shown that there was no much difference in hydrolysis rate of medium chain or of longer chain fatty acid. I wonder if the explanation could possibly be due to the fact that if you have a triglyceride, you must orient the triglyceride at the surface of the globule and I've assumed that the fatty acids that are orientated towards the surface could be the short chain fatty acids, the medium chain fatty acids and the polyunsaturated fatty acids. Wouldn't you expect these fatty acids to be hydrolysed first?

M. Hamosh: Well, you would expect but it's nice when you find it.

O. Hernell: But I think there may be a preference for the substrate but I think that you can show that if you have the triglyceride then you have.

M. Hamosh: Well, see for the lingual and gastric you have a positional specificity in such a way that you can put the most preferential fatty acid in the wrong position and nothing will happen. I agree with you that a lot of what happens in lipids is orientation at the interphase with the medium chain ones, the short chain ones and the long chain polyunsaturated of course being more water micellable and they will be attacked first, but I'm surprised to see however that if you incubate for quite a long time both *in vivo* and *in vitro* the long chain saturated do not budge or budge to a very low extent. Maybe we will have a way to modify what mother eats for the breast fed infant and what the formula company puts in, because maybe having all those (especially for the premature infant) palmitic or stearic triglyceride might not be the best idea because they are just sitting there.

M. Vidailhet: Another question: What is calculated at 62% of hydrolysis? Is that 62% of the total ester bonds of triglycerides?

M. Hamosh: Exactly that's what it is, it's a lot of hydrolysis.

C. Galli: Human gastric lipase is extremely sensitive to fatty acid inhibition. Did you expect this 62% hydrolysis?

M. Hamosh: This was for the dog and we are now looking at some other ingredients in dog milk. For the human we find easily 30% hydrolysis but in the dog if you wait for 60 min, you find 60% hydrolysis.

C. Galli: What's about the value when you took the samples at different times and calculated the composition, that was the composition of what was left in the stomach?

M. Hamosh: We do it in three ways; we first analyse the sample we have at O time which is the milk composition as far as total fatty acids triglyceride fatty acids and free fatty acids. Then we aspired at different time interval and we do the same analysis, total fatty acids, triglycerides, fatty acids and free fatty acids.

M. Vidailhet: I did not see in your very detailed composition of milk fat, very long chain fatty acid C24, C26 and so on, are they totally absent?

M. Hamosh: I have shown the 22:6 and 22:5 in human milk which in our population, tested around 1982-1983, were not very high, because the American diet was not very high in those fatty acids, and I don't know to what extent they are produced in the mammary gland; however if you look at the dog data, the dog just does not have those fatty acids, it does not have a trace of them and we have looked many, many times, so it is part of the dog diet and we are also analysing the dog diet; so there is what mamma eats and mum does not desaturate anymore. We are however going to look at what happens in the mammary gland.

Chairman: Last question.

C. Galli: I would like to ask you if you can tell us the mechanism as possible for the dramatic fall in cholesterol and phospholipid content, and if there is an associated change with the particle size or with the structure of the membrane.

M. Hamosh: It is definitely associated with particle sizes but I think that particle size is the first thing and the second thing is that the mammary gland becomes much more efficient. It learns within ten days how to package and in the beginning packaging is very inefficient; it makes more globules and uses a lot of its own membranes to package them; within two weeks it becomes a perfect packager and makes much bigger globules which contain much more triglycerides and they need much less membrane to hold them inside; what is the exact mechanism, whether there are changes in the availability of cholesterol and in the availability of phospholipids for this process I don't know if anybody has looked at that.

C. Galli: What about the efficiency of the lipase on the different globules; is that depending on the size and is it modified with the time?

M. Hamosh: Well, I would expect that pancreatic lipase doesn't know what to do with fat globules, but lingual and gastric can penetrate the phospholipid layer very easily so they can go in; if the layer is thicker and they have then more problem to be penetrated, I don't know.

B. Koletzko: If I may make a comment on that it is always a question of the surface pressure of the globule which may be modified with human milk protein, pancreatic lipase.

M. Hamosh: But I think what he has shown is very interesting also from the point of view that a lot of it is *in vitro* work and I don't know whether the milk fat globules will behave in exactly the same way but what has been done is taking emulsions and taking those proteins which are present in milk in different concentrations but we all know that those you can get a lot of arte factual observations, not arte factual because it is what happens *in vitro*; whether the same thing happens *in vivo*, whether the packaging of the globule is exactly the same as adding the protein from the outside or adding the phospholipid from the outside or adding cholesterol from the outside is really not known.

Chairman: So I would like to thank very, very much the two speakers for their very interesting lectures and also the audience for the pertinent questions.

SESSION VI

Round table

Chairman: Jean REY (France)

13

How to appreciate an inadequate essential fatty acid intake in infancy

J. GHISOLFI

Service de Médecine Infantile D, CHU Purpan, Hôpital de Purpan, Place du Docteur-Baylac, 31059 Toulouse Cedex, France

Considering infant nutrition in clinical practice, the current problem is no more to cure an essential fatty acid (EFA) deficiency status. It is today to estimate what must be the optimal essential fatty acid intake to prevent any deleterious effect on growth, development, membrane functions, eicosanoid synthesis. For evident ethical considerations, this estimation is not easy in babies.

Several approaches can be used as a measure of the adequacy of n–6 and n–3 fatty acids in infant diets.

An inadequate EFA intake is difficult to evaluate through clinical data. If we do not consider the particular symptoms resulting from severe essential fatty acid deficiency supplies, which include growth retardation, scaly dermatitis, increased transepidermal water loss, any clinical sign is characteristic of a non-optimal EFA supply. Many thousands of full-term and premature infants have grown well without recognised clinical evidence of any nutritional troubles with diets containing less than 0.5% of kilocalories as linoleic acid (LA) and less of 0.1% of kilocalories as alphalinolenic acid (ALA). There is apparently no clinical differences certainly linked to EFA intakes between breast-fed babies and formula-fed infants. Clinical consequences of a very insufficient alphalinolenic acid intake have only been recognised in children during long term artificial nutrition and never in normal infants fed usual formulas. Increased transepidermal water loss is a well documented linoleic acid deficiency symptom in infants. Using a servomed evaporimeter which allows a direct quantitative water evaporation measurement, we could observe this increase of water evaporation in very severe EFA deficiency status, but we did not note any correlation between skin water loss and various LA intakes from 0.3% to 15% of kilocalories as LA in normal babies. It may be concluded that an inadequate essential fatty acid intake higher than 1.0% for linoleic acid and higher than 0.3% for alphalinolenic acid of total kilocalories cannot probably be evaluated through usual clinical data.

Because of their accessibility blood samples have often been used to appreciate essential fatty acid status in infancy. Plasma fatty acids have been said to mimic dietary fats. Total plasma fatty acid determination is usually performed rather than analysis of individual lipid classes. As many other authors, we have observed that fatty acid percentages of plasma total lipids change in relation to dietary lipids. However, plasma phospholipids contain the major fraction of plasma polyunsaturated FA and because they are less likely to be influenced by exogenous triglycerides, they are potentially a more occurate indicators of EFA intake than is total serum lipids or serum triglycerides and cholesteryl ester fractions. But individual serum phospholipids vary widely in their response to linoleic or linolenic acid intake variations. So, it is certainly necessary to separate the phospholipids from lipid extract of the serum and to analyse fatty acid percentage changes in the different phospholipids: phosphatidylcholine (PC), phosphatidyl ethanolamine (PE), phosphatidyl inositol (PI) and serine (PS). Biochemical diagnosis of essential fatty acid deficiency is most often based on analysis of relative percentage of each fatty acid, in total or individual plasma phospholipids, particularly $C18 = 2$ n–6, $C20 = 4$ n–6, $C20 = 3$ n–9 (triene: tetraene ratio). Considering variations of linoleic acid intakes from 1% to 8% of total kilocalories in normal fed infants, we observed an increase of linoleic acid percentage in phosphatidyl ethanolamine and phosphatidyl choline, but rather a decrease of dihomogammalinolenic and arachidonic acids. But this approach does not occurately allow to appreciate the n–6 or n–3 fatty acid status of the different organs in relation to lipid diets. The fatty acid composition of plasma phospholipid is influenced by dietary intake, but also by preferential tissue uptake, specific fatty acid metabolism and possibly beta oxydation, particularly in protein energy malnutrition status. Additional valuable information could possibly be obtained by indicating the fatty acid quantitative changes which occur in individual plasma phospholipids, triglycerides or cholesteryl ester fractions, but little information exists on the adequacy of this approach because most authors express their fatty acid data as a relative percent of the total FA and not as in absolute concentration (micromol/l plasma). In conclusion, it is therefore certain that plasma phospholipid fatty acid distribution depends on dietary fatty acids but probably does not reflect exact fatty acid tissue status in relation to changes in lipid supplies.

Effects of variations in dietary fatty acid on erythrocyte membrane phospholipids in infants is now well investigated. Comparative analyses of the fatty acid composition of red blood cell glycerophospholipids among infants fed various formulas or breast milks have been used as a measure of the adequacy of essential fatty acids, particularly of n–3 fatty acids, in infant diets. As many other authors we observed a significant correlation between linoleic acid supplies and linoleic acid percentages in erythrocyte phospholipids. Possibly more important, erythrocyte long-chain polyenoates (LCP) can be influenced by dietary fatty acids. In human infants, red blood cell LCP of the n–3 family are decreased and those of the n–6 family increased with the feeding of an increased dietary ratio of $C18 = 2$ n–6/$C18 = 3$ n–3. It is now demonstrated that the dietary ratio of LA/ALA in diet influences erythrocyte membrane concentration of n–6 and n–3 metabolites. As commercial formulas available today derive their fat from a variety of vegetable oils which do not provide any 20 to 22 carbon polyunsaturated fatty acids, feeding infants with these formulas results in significantly lower erythrocyte membrane concentrations of the long-chain polyunsaturates of both the n–3 and n–6 families, compared to those receiving human milk. Percentages of C20 = 5 n–3 and C22 = 6 n–3 are increased in erythrocyte phospholipids when fish oils containing n–3 LCP are added to their formulas and are similar to the levels noted in breast milk-fed infants. Therefore, it can be concluded that the levels of LCP in red blood cell phospholipids reflect the quality of lipids absorbed from diet. However little variations from 1 to 5% acids as linoleic and/or alphalinolenic acid do not result in notable differences in erythrocyte n–6 or n–3 LCP. But it has been also observed that erythrocyte glycerophospholipid n–6 and n–3 LCP, particularly C20 = 4 n–6 and C22 = 6 n–3 are lower in very prematurate infants than in term infants when either formula or breast milk is used as the source of nutrition. These data certainly require consideration, particularly if, as it has been shown in piglets, there is a direct correlation between fatty acid composition of red blood cells and brain membrane phospholipids. On the basis of these data, it has been suggested that erythrocyte lipid dosages may be used to evaluate n–3 LCP status of brain and retina, but today it is not certain that comparative analyses of red blood cell LCP may offer a specific measure of LCP status in organs. Probably, diet-induced changes in the fatty acid composition of lipid erythrocytes do not fully reflect changes in the fatty acid composition of organs such as liver, brain and retina, which are capable of *in situ* fatty acid desaturation and elongation. The fatty acids of the mature red cells are continually modified by deacylation and reacylation with plasma fatty acids and by exchange with plasma phospholipids. On the other hand, organs, and particularly brain, are more resistant to dietary fatty acids manipulations than are erythrocytes. Furthermore, it has been shown by Lefkowhith *et al.*, on mice, that each organ, differently responds to variations in lipid diets. The data observed by these authors suggest that the liver serves to supply other tissues with arachidonate in EFA deficiency status. Today however, even if red blood cell phospholipid composition does not occurately reflect the fatty acid concentrations in organs of infants, this type of analysis remains very used. Perhaps, as for plasma phospholipids, rather than relative percentage of total fatty acid, quantitative expression is worth thinking over and studying.

In conclusion, it is certain that red blood cell phospholipid fatty acid distribution depends on dietary fatty acids but our present knowledge probably does not allow us to consider that fatty acid composition of red blood cell phospholipids can be used as an index of LCP status. Fatty acid variations in erythrocytes do not allow an exact estimation of the consequences of diet on the fatty acid composition on the other organs.

Autopsy and *in vivo* organ biopsy studies have shown without doubt that tissue concentration of membrane long-chain polyenoates can be influenced by dietary fatty acids. But evidently, in normal infants for ethical reasons, it is not possible to obtain tissue samples. Certain samples can be however easely taken. For instance, analysis of the fatty acid composition of phospholipids in human cheeks (buccal epithelial cells) has been suggested as a non-invasive method for monitoring the fatty acid composition of diets in adult humans. This tissue with rapid turnover was speculated to be more likely to reflect current diet than either erythrocytes or fat stores. We have had the opportunity to confirm this fact on cheek cells which were collected in babies by scraping the cheek mucosa with a spoon. As it has been shown in adults, we noted in infants a good correlation between linoleic acid concentration in cheek cell total phospholipids and linoleic acid intake. However this correlation only appeared after two months of diet. It becomes only significant with very important differences in linoleic acid intake from 2-5 to 10% of total kilocalories. The percentage of arachidonic acid was also slightly modified. We did not observe any correlation between alphalinolenic acid intake and n–3 LCP percentage in cheek cell phospholipids. Using our methodology, according to the very little quantity of cheek cells we can obtain in babies, analysis of the fatty acid composition of cheek cell phospholipids does not appear as available, except perhaps to evaluate linoleic acid intake. On this point, it is interesting to note that we observed a good correlation between linoleic and arachidonic acids in erythrocyte and cheek cell phospholipids.

Diet fat composition also influences the adipose tissue membrane fatty acid composition and this may alter the structure and functional properties of adipocyte membrane. However structural lipids in human adipose tissue seem more resistant to changes in relation to fat diet than stored triglycerides. We studied the fatty acid distribution in adipocyte membrane phospholipids in infant receiving various linoleic acid intakes. Adipose tissue samples were obtained during abdominal surgical procedures for therapeutic reasons. We observed a good correlation ($p < 0.01$) between linoleic acid intake and linoleic or arachidonic acids in adipocyte membrane phospholipids but this correlation only appeared when using very different amounts of linoleic acid intake from 300 mg to 1500 mg/kg/24 h and after at least one or two months of defined diets. It is to note that we also found a correlation concerning linoleic and arachidonic acid between erythrocyte and membrane adipose tissue phospholipids ($p < 0.05$). But in any case, these fatty acid composition variations in two tissues do not allow an estimation of the consequences on the fatty acid distribution of the other organs. It is well known that each tissue and lipid class responds differently to change in fat regimen.

It is therefore demonstrated that membrane fatty acid composition varies with fat diet. But except in very particular conditions, as in infants who only received total parenteral nutrition and died during the neonatal period, there is very little information on the effects of dietary lipids variations on fatty acid tissue composition.

Insufficient knowledge of how lipid diet content affects membrane function makes changes in tissue lipid composition of little value, except as an index of dietary fat quality and quantity. For instance, in the conditions of various linoleic or alphalinolenic acid intake as it is observed in formula-fed or breast-fed infants, really no clear relationship between fatty acid composition and membrane fluidity has been demonstrated. We do not have any data which show that these changes in tissue phospholipid fatty acid distribution, linked to the difference in fatty acid composition of formulas, may affect physiological functions (physical properties, enzyme activities, receptor functions) in normal babies. However polyenoic fatty acids are major structural components of specialized neuronal membranes. Visual alteration and altered learning behavior have been described in association with n–6 or n–3 fatty acid variations in the diet. Non-specific visual changes and peripheral neuropathy have been observed in chronically ill patients on a free alphalinolenic acid artificial nutrition in humans. Recently it has been reported by Uauy *et al.* improved visual evoked potential acuity in very low-birth-weight infants fed different marine oil supplemented and control non-marine oil supplemented formulas. These data seem to demonstrate that n–3 fatty acids are essential for optimal function of the developing retina. Certainly, these approaches using electroretinogram and evoked potential are to be developed particularly for premature infants, to appreciate effects of n–3 LCP variations in diets on growing brain and retina.

Triglyceride stores in adipose tissue are strongly correlated to linoleic acid intake in infancy. Because of the rapid growth and turnover of adipose tissue in infants, this correlation is particularly noted at this age. In several studies on babies receiving for at least two months various fat regimen, we observed that white adipose tissue accumulates linoleic, dihomogammalinolenic and arachidonic acids in significant relation to linoleic acid intake and $C18 = 3$ n–3, $C22 = 6$ n–3 in relation to alphalinolenic linolenic intake. This fact is probably of nutritional importance as, at this stage of life, the infants build up their EFA stores.

Eicosanoid synthesis is linked to n–6 and n–3 LCP membrane content. In our knowledge we do not have any study on the effect of changes in EFA supply on tissue eicosanoid synthesis. We only know that the prostaglandin urinary excretion rates are related to linoleic acid intake. We observed in infants this correlation but only when we used an amount of linoleic acid intake lower than recommended requirements (150 mg/kg/24h). Above 350 mg/kg/24h, the prostaglandins urinary excretion does not significantly change in normal infants. Diet certainly modifies prostaglandin urinary excretion but probably does not affect eicosanoid tissue synthesis, except in severe essential fatty acid deficiency status. The generation of free arachidonic acid and n–3 LCP from membrane phospholipids is probably sufficient to maintain eicosanoid synthesis upon various physiological or pathological stimuli. Prostaglandin urinary excretion cannot be used to estimate optimal essential fatty acid requirements, but probably can be used to evaluate insufficient essential fatty acid intakes.

The n–6 and n–3 LCP synthesis is primarily dependent on the activity of the desaturase enzymes. It has been observed that administration of relatively high contents of $CF18 = 2$ n–6 in formulas reduced levels of arachidonic acid, polyunsaturated fatty acids with 22 carbons, and prostaglandin synthesis in infants receiving total parenteral nutrition. Experimental data, *in vitro* or *in vivo* studies, show that large dietary excess of different fatty acids as $C18 = 1$ n–9, $C18 = 2$ n–6, $C18 = 3$ n–3 or n–3 LCP, interfere with desaturation system and can inhibit n–6 or n–3 LCP synthesis. This question is important to debate as it moots the question of adverse effects of high linoleic, alphalinolenic acids, or marine oil intakes. Studies of fatty acid variations on membrane phospholipids as erythrocytes allow to evaluate the consequences of changes in essential fatty supplies on desaturase activities. In a study in normal full-term babies receiving large variations of linoleic acid supplies, from 150 to 2000 mg/kg/24 h, we noted in relation to increase of linoleic acid intake a significant increase of linoleic acid in erythrocyte, cheek cells, adipose membrane phospholipids, in triglyceride adipose tissue, and never a decrease of the higher homologues of $C18 = 2$ n–6 and $C18 = 3$ n–3, particularly of $C20 = 4$ n–6 and $C22 = 6$ n–3. The effects of high EFA or LCP intakes are probably different and patent in very critically ill babies and in premature infants.

It may be concluded that if it is easy to recognise clinical or biochemical signs of essential fatty acid deficiency, it is difficult today to really evaluate the clinical, biochemical and functional consequences of an inadequate essential fatty acid intake in infancy. Our approach is not precise enough and does not permit a good estimation of optimal essential fatty acid requirements. However we have to consider with attention the experimental data and the actual knowledge on fatty acid changes in organs, or on specific fatty acid accumulation on tissues as brain and retina particularly during the growing period and their functional consequences which begin to be appreciated.

14

Minimal, optimal, maximal essential fatty acid requirements during infancy: term infants

B. KOLETZKO

Kinderklinik der Heinrich-heine-Universität, Moorenstr 5,
D-4000 Düsseldorf 1, Germany

Presently the essential fatty acid requirements of healthy human infants cannot be exactly defined. Too little data are available on the effects of different quantities of dietary essential fatty acids on body composition and function in full term infants. Also, it is probably not possible to draw a sharp line between a sufficient and a deficient essential fatty acid intake, since nutrient supply may be at any point of a continuous spectrum from deficient to excessive and possibly even toxic levels (*figure 1*). Several factors may alter requirements in individuals and shift this distribution curve up- or downwards. Such variables may include individual factors such as intrauterine nutrient supply, body weight, age, growth rate and possibly genetic factors, environmental conditions such as ambient temperature and humidity, metabolic and endocrine factors, and composition of diet [1] (*Table I*). Since the optimal essential fatty acid intake of term infants cannot be defined with certainty at present, one has to make rather pragmatic decisions on desirable ranges of intakes that can be expected, with a certain margin of safety, to prevent known and suspected untoward effects of deficient or excessive intakes in formula fed infants. Two major questions are to be addressed (1) which essential fatty acids should be supplied to the neonate; and (2) what quantities and ratios of individual fatty acids and fatty acid families appear desirable?

Table I. Some factors that may alter essential fatty acid requirements in infants

Individual factors Intrauterine supply and body stores at birth, postconceptional and postnatal age, body weight, growth rate, stress, trauma, infection, genetic factors?
Environmental conditions Temperature, humidity
Metabolic factors Lipid and eicosanoid metabolism and turnover, enzyme and receptor activity, energy expenditure and energy balance, rate of fat oxidation
Endocrine factors Insulin, glucagon, adrenalin, cortisol, thyroxin
Dietary components Intakes of energy, protein, carbohydrates, cholesterol, saturated fats, trans-isomeric fats, medium-chain fatty acids, zinc, copper, selenium, nucleotides, tocopherol, retinol

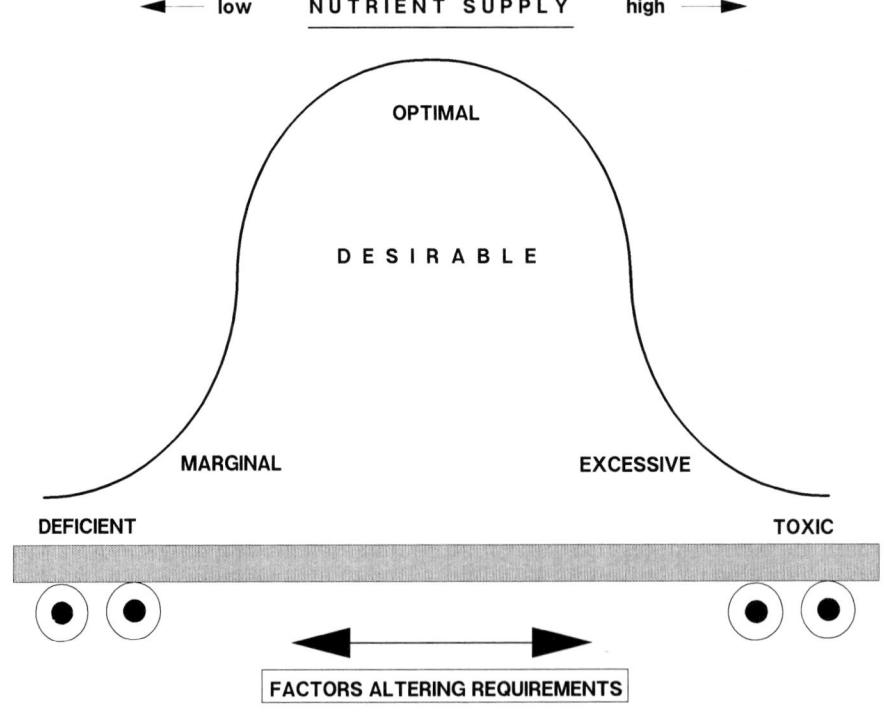

Figure 1. Continuous spectrum of nutrient ranging from deficient to toxic levels. Several factors may alter requirements in individuals and, thereby, shift the distribution curve up- or downwards.

Linoleic acid requirements

In the past, linoleic acid (C18:2n-6)* was considered the only fatty acid that has to be supplied with the diet. Official recommendations on the essential fatty acid composition of infant formulas for full term babies used to be restricted to figures on the linoleic acid content (*Table II*). Most expert committees gave only recommendations on the lower limit of linoleic intakes ranging from 1 to 3% of energy intakes. Only recently the Commission of the European Communities and the Committee on Nutrition of the European Society for Paediatric Gastroenterology and Nutrition (ESPGAN) recommended an upper limit for linoleic acid of 10.8% of energy intake. Previously, no recommendations were given for any other essential fatty acid or ratio with respect to full term infants. The only exception is the new guideline of the ESPGAN Committee on Nutrition which recommended also a supply of the omega-3 fatty acid alpha-linolenic acid [26].

Table II. Recommendations on the essential fatty acid intake of mature newborn infants

Linoleic acid intake	Recommending body
≥ 2 energy %	US Food and Drug Administration 1971
≥ 2.7 energy %	American Academy of Pediatrics 1976
≥ 2.7 energy %	FAO/WHO Codex Alimentarius 1976
≥ 3 energy %^{2}	ESPGAN Committee on Nutrition 1977
≥ 1 energy %	Committee Medical Aspects Food Policy 1980
≥ 2.7 energy % ≤ 10.8 energy %	Commission European Communities 1991
≥ 2.7 energy % ≤ 10.8 energy %^{3}	ESPGAN Committee on Nutrition 1991

^{2} A range of 3-6 energy % was suggested but no upper limit was set.
^{3} In addition, a linoleic/alpha-linolenic acid ratio in the range from 5 to 15 was recommended.

The previous recommendations aimed primarily at the prevention of the linoleic acid deficiency syndrome. Full term infants fed for a period of about 2 to 3 months a formula diet practically devoid of fat develop a failure to thrive, an increased susceptibility to infections and a typical scaly dermatitis [1-3]. The minimal amount of essential fatty acids required to prevent these symptoms is not exactly known. However, we have some information on the dimension of essential fatty acid requirements from the early work of Hansen *et al.* [3]. These investigators induced dietary linoleic acid deficiency in term and preterm infants, and the occuring symptoms were cured in single infants with a supply of butterfat providing about 1.3% of energy intake as linoleic acid. It appears possible that even lower intakes of linoleic acid might be effective but this was not tested by Hansen *et al.* On the other hand, butterfat contains not only linoleic acid but also small amounts of its long chain metabolites which have a higher essential fatty acid activity than linoleic

---

* Conventionally, short formulas are used to describe fatty acids. They denote the number of carbon atoms in the acyl chain, the number of double bonds, and in case of an unsaturated fatty acid the position of the terminal double bond (e.g. C18:2n-6 for linoleic acid, C18:3n-3 for alpha-linolenic acid).

acid, and the cure of human essential fatty acid deficiency with 1.3% energy of pure linoleic acid was not demonstrated. Alpha-linolenic acid (C18:3n-3) has also been used to cure the deficiency syndrome, but its therapeutic effect on dermal deficiency symptoms in animals is low and equivalent to only about one tenth of the effect of linoleic acid [4].

However, the generally accepted conclusion from Hansen's studies was that a dietary linoleic acid intake in the order of 1.3% of energy intake would be sufficient to prevent occurrence of essential fatty acid deficiency.

In addition to the use of clinical symptoms, attempts have been made to define human essential fatty acid requirements on the basis of certain biochemical markers. It has been proposed that definition of adequate essential fatty acid intakes could be delineated from the composition of blood plasma lipids, specifically from the ratio of Mead acid (C20:3n-9) to arachidonic acid (C20:4n-6). Mead acid is derived from the non-essential oleic acid (C18:1n-9) by further desaturation and chain-elongation in a complex microsomal enzyme system (*figure 2*). Linoleic (C18:2n-6) and alpha-linolenic acid (C18:3n-3) bind to the same enzyme system with a much higher affinitiy, and they inhibit competitively the desaturation of oleic acid. Therefore, little Mead acid is synthetized from oleic acid unless dietary intake and intracellular concentrations of linoleic and alpha-linolenic acids are very low.

An expert committee of the United Nations Food and Agricultural Organization stated in 1980 that a ratio of Mead to arachidonic acid greater than 0.2 in serum lipids would indicate essential fatty acid deficiency [5]. This conclusion was based mainly on data from animal studies. The use of this ratio is quite attractive because it reflects intracellular metabolism. On the other hand, the ratio may be influenced by factors other than linoleic acid intake, such as availability of oleic acid from diet, endogenous synthesis and body stores, and the activity levels of the desaturating and chain elongating enzymes which may be low in infancy. Moreover, it is not

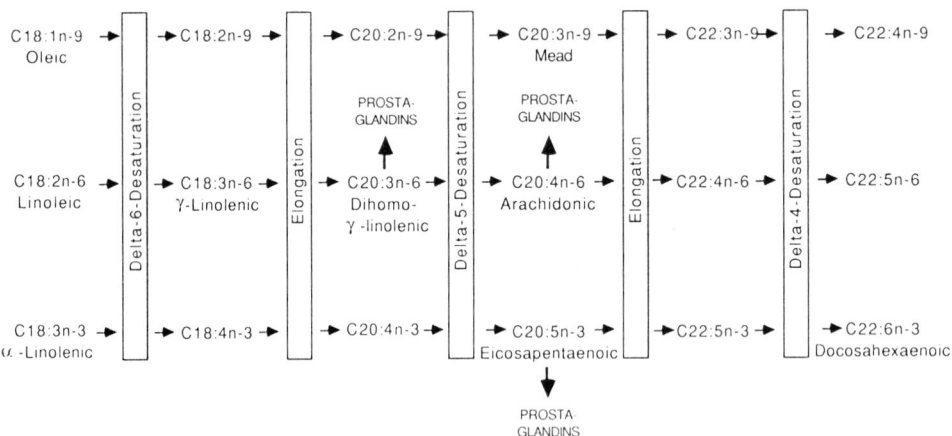

Figure 2. Metabolism of unsaturated fatty acids. Fatty acids of the n-9 (omega 9), n-6 (omega 6) and n-3 (omega 3) compete for one system of several microsomal enzymes for further desaturation and chain-elongation. (Reproduced from Koletzko B. Fats for brains. *Eur J Clin Nutr*, in press).

clear to which extent other fatty acids such as the long-chain products of linoleic and alpha-linolenic acids may influence the Mead acid/arachidonic acid ratio. Overall, there is no hard evidence that in human infants a value of 0.2 for this ratio would be an appropriate threshold level above which clinical deficiency symptoms will occur.

In conclusion, neither the available reports on clinically symptomatic essential fatty acid deficiency and its cure nor the studies measuring the Mead acid/arachidonic acid ratio allow to clearly define the minimal linoleic acid requirements of the human infant. However, in practice this is not a problem at all because we do not need or want to feed only the minimal amount of linoleic acid.

Maximal intake of linoleic acid

The guidelines of the European Communities [6] and of the Committee on Nutrition of the European Society for Paediatric Gastroenterology and Nutrition [26] recommend that linoleic acid should not contribute more than 10.8% of energy in infant formulas. This cautious approach was chosen in view of potential side effects of high dietary intakes of polyunsaturated fatty acids, even though little evidence on actual side effects in infants is available.

In the 1970ies, a large number of infants in the Netherlands was fed a formula with all dietary fat provided by corn oil [7]. In this formula linoleic acid contributed almost 60% of all dietary fatty acids, while there were only minor amounts of alpha-linolenic acid. Although no clinical side effects were reported, Widdowson et al. demonstrated marked effects on tissue composition in infants. Feeding of the linoleic acid rich formula resulted in a remarkable enrichment of linoleic acid in adipose tissue. It is not known to which extent other tissues and membrane structures were altered in their composition, and how this may have affected membrane functions and activities of membrane bound receptors and enzymes. Widdowson also noted that infants receiving the high linoleic acid intakes had low serum cholesterol values. It is not known whether this reduction of circulating cholesterol may affect cholesterol deposition in growing membranes and the extent of cholesterol conversion to steroid hormones.

Other possible side effects of high linoleic acid intakes are decreases in the tissue concentrations of its major metabolite arachidonic acid (C20:4n-6) and disturbed prostaglandin turnover, as documented both in human adults [8] and infants [9].

Furthermore, very high intakes of linoleic acid were shown to act immunosuppressive and to inhibit cell mediated immunity, inflammatory reactions and thymic weight as well as the synthesis of complement and immunoglobulins [10-12]. Since the newborn infant has an immature immune system and is highly prone to infections, a significant additional suppression of immune and inflammatory reactions by an extremely high dietary supply of polyunsaturated fatty acids would be undesirable.

Of particular concern is the risk of adverse effects of enhanced lipid peroxidation and generation of free radicals with nutritional products that are very high in polyunsaturated fatty acids [13]. In animal experiments, free radicals and lipid peroxides damage proteins, enzymes, membrane structures, and even DNA, and they can disrupt the integrity of intestinal mucosa and produce diarrhea, growth retardation and death [14, 15]. In newborn infants, intravenous infusion of linoleic acid rich lipids results in enhanced peroxide formation and exhalation of ethane and pentane [16]. Also, the requirements of antioxidants such as tocopherols increase with increasing dietary intakes of polyunsaturated fatty acids [17, 18].

In view of the potential untoward effects of high intakes of polyunsaturates, it appears prudent to avoid extremely high contents of linoleic acid and other polyunsaturated fatty acids in infant formulas.

Alpha-linolenic acid

The second major essential fatty acid in vegetable oils is alpha-linolenic acid (C18:3n-3) of the omega-3 series. Although occurence of a specific alpha-linolenic acid deficiency with typical symptoms has been proposed [19, 20], the evidence has been questioned [21-23]. There is no indication that alpha-linolenic acid itself has any essential structural roles. In fact, the oxidation of alpha-linolenic acid in rodents is higher than that of any other unsaturated fatty acids [24] suggesting that its biological value for the organism is not very high. However, alpha-linolenic acid is the substrate for the synthesis of omega-3 long-chain polyunsaturated fatty acids (LCP) such as docosahexaenoic acid (C22:6n-3) (*figure 2*) that certainly have essential functions in brain and retina [25]. Moreover, alpha-linolenic acid competes with linoleic acid for the formation of n-6 and n-3 LCP. In animals, the dietary linoleic/alpha-linolenic acid-ratio modulates not only tissue contents of n-6 and n-3 LCP but also the function of brain and retina (Koletzko, in press). Therefore, it appears preferable to avoid extreme linoleic/alpha-linolenic acid ratios in infant formulas. The ESPGAN Committee on Nutrition [26] recommended that in infant formula lipids the linoleic/alpha-linolenic acid ratio should be in the range from 5 to 15, which is similar to typical human milk values.

Long-chain polyunsaturated fatty acids

Long-chain polyunsaturated fatty acids with 20 and 22 carbon atoms (LCP), such as arachidonic acid (C20:4n-6) of the omega-6 series and docosahexaenoic acid (C22:6n-3) of the omega-3 series, are derived from linoeic and alpha-linolenic acids (*figure 2*). Relatively large amounts of n-6 and n-3 LCP are deposited during late foetal and early postnatal growth in the developing brain, retina and other tissues. There is accumulating evidence that the availability of n-6 and n-3 LCP during the perinatal period modulates tissue growth and the development of neural and retinal functions [37, 25]. Prenatally, n-6 and n-3 LCP are preferentially transferred from the mother to the foetus by selective placental transport mechanisms [36]. Postnatally, human milk lipids provide sufficient amounts of n-6 and n-3 LCP to breast fed infants to meet all LCP requirements for tissue deposition [22, 25]. In contrast, current infant formulas do not contain appreciable amounts of LCP [27]. We found no docosahexaenoic acid in any of 25 infant formulas sold in Germany, and only a few formulas had small amounts of arachidonic acid apparently originating from butterfat (*Table III*). Full term and especially premature infants fed such formula with linoleic and alpha-linolenic acids but without LCP develop depletion of n-6 and n-3 LCP in plasma and membrane lipids to values significantly lower than in infants fed human milk [28-31]. In premature infants, LCP depletion has been related to functional abnormalities such as impaired visual acuity [25, 32, 33]. Therefore, the Committee of Nutrition of ESPGAN considered enrichment of formulas for low birthweight infants with n-6 and n-3 LCP desirable in order to prevent LCP depletion of infantile structural lipids and their possible functional consequences [26]. For infants born at term it is presently not known whether they may also benefit from a dietary LCP supply with formulas, and no such recommendation has been issued.

Table III. Essential fatty acids (% wt/wt) in mature human milk (n = 15, adapted from Koletzko *et al.* 1988) and 25 infant formulas sold in Germany (adapted from Koletzko *et al.*, 1989)

	Human milk	Formulas
	Median ± IQR	Median (Range)
Linoleic acid (C18:2n-6)	10.8 ± 1.1	12.3 (9.0-53.5)
Alpha-linolenic acid (C18:3n-3)	0.8 ± 0.2	0.7 (0.4-2.4)
Arachidonic (C20:4n-6)	0.4 ± 0.0	0.0 (0.0-0.2)
Docosahexaenoic (C22:6n-3)	0.2 ± 0.1	0.0 (0.0-0.0)

Composition of human milk lipids as a model for infant formulas

The optimal amounts and relative ratios of different fatty acids which are associated with the best short and long term outcome cannot be determined at present. Therefore, the fatty acid composition of human milk is often used as a reference model for infant formulas. This approach has been questioned because fatty acid patterns of human milk may vary with the diet of lactating women. We recently studied the extent of this variation and reviewed reports on the fatty acid composition of mature human milk from 9 European (14 studies) and 7 African countries (10 studies) [34]. In spite of marked differences in the methodology used in the various studies and the great variation of dietary composition in different parts of Europe and Africa, average essential fatty acid results are surprisingly consistent (*Table IV*). The diet of lactating women apparently influences, to a limited extent, human milk content of saturated and monounsaturated fatty acids and of linoleic acid (C18:2n-6). In contrast, milk LCP seem relatively little affected by geographic variation of self

Table IV. Essential fatty acids in mature human milk in 14 European and 10 African studies (% wt/wt, median values and ranges. Adapted from Koletzko et al., J Pediatr, in press)

	Europe	Africa
N-6 PUFA:		
C18:2n-6 (linoleic)	11.0 (6.9-16.4)	12.0 (5.7-17.2)
C20:2n-6	0.3 (0.2-0.5)	0.3 (0.3-0.8)
C20:3n-6	0.3 (0.2-0.7)	0.4 (0.2-0.5)
C20:4n-6 (arachidonic)	0.5 (0.2-1.2)	0.6 (0.3-1.0)
C22:4n-6	0.1 (0.1-0.2)	0.1 (0.0-0.1)
C22:5n-6	0.1 (0.0-0.2)	0.1 (0.1-0.3)
Total n-6 LCP	1.2 (0.4-2.2)	1.5 (0.9-2.0)
N-3 PUFA:		
C18:3n-3 (a-linolenic)	0.9 (0.7-1.3)	0.8 (0.1-1.4)
C20:5n-3 (eicospentaenoic)	0.2 (0.0-0.6)	0.1 (0.1-0.5)
C22:5n-3	0.2 (0.1-0.5)	0.2 (0.1-0.4)
C22:6n-3 (docosahexaenoic)	0.3 (0.1-0.6)	0.3 (0.1-0.9)
Total n-3 LCP	0.6 (0.3-1.8)	0.6 (0.3-2.9)
Ratios		
Ratio 18:2n-6/18:3n-3	12.1 (8.6-16.9)	14.2 (8.8-157)
Ratio 20:4n-6/22:6n-3	1.8 (0.7-5.0)	2.2 (0.7-10)
Ratio n-6 LCP/n-3LCP	2.7 (0.3-3.7)	2.4 (0.8-6)

selected diets. Rural African women consuming little animal fat tend to have high milk contents of n-6 LCP, thus the LCP secretion in milk does not depend on maternal dietary intake of preformed LCP [35]. We conclude that in addition to the composition of maternal diet, metabolic processes regulate the essential fatty acid content of human milk. It is tempting to speculate that such regulatory processes may represent a protective mechanism for the infant providing a relatively constant dietary supply of physiologically important fatty acids. Given our current deficits in understanding the metabolism and the effects of dietary fatty acids in infants, it appears prudent to obtain some orientation from the biological model of human milk composition when designing lipid compositions of infant formulas, even though there is no scientific basis to directly deduct fatty acid requirements of the human infant from average composition of human milk. There may still be some truth in the 19th century statement of Oliver Wendell Holmes (1809-1894): "A pair of substantial mammary glands have the advantage over the two hemispheres of the most learned professor's brain in the art of compounding a nutritive fluid for infants."

Acknowledgement

The work of the author is financially supported by Deutsche Forschungsgemeinschaft, Bonn, Germany (Ko 912/1-1 and Ko 912/4-1).

References

1. Koletzko B. (1986) Essentielle Fettsäuren: Bedeutung für Medizin und Ernährung. *Aktuel Endokr Stoffw* 7:18-27.
2. Von Groer F. (1919) Zur Frage des praktischen Bedeutung des Nährwertbegriffes nebst einigen Bemerkungen über das Fettminimum des menschlichen Säuglings. *Biochem Z* 97:311-29.
3. Hansen A.E., Wiese H.F., Boelsche A.N., Haggard M.E., Adam D.J.D., Davis H. (1963) Role of linoleic acid in infant nutrition. *Pediatrics* 31:171-92.
4. Thomasson H.J. (1953) Biological standardization of essential fatty acids (a new method). *Int J Vitamin Nutr Res* 25:62-82.
5. Food and Agriculture Organization of the United Nations (1980) Dietary fats and oils in human nutrition. FAO, Publications Division, Rome.
6. Commission of the European Communities (1991) Directorate-General, Internal Market and Industrial Affairs. Commission Directive on infant formulae and follow-on formulae. Brussels, Commission of the European Communities.
7. Widdowson E.M. (1989) Upper limits of intakes of total fat and polyunsaturated fatty acids in infant formulas. *J Nutr* 119:1814-7.
8. Adam O., Wolfram G. (1984) Effect of different linoleic acid intakes on prostaglandin biosynthesis and kidney function in man. *Am J Clin Nutr* 40:763-70.
9. Friedman Z., Frölich J.C. (1979) Essential fatty acids and the major urinary metabolites of the E prostaglandins in thriving neonates and in infants receiving parenteral fat emulsions. *Pediatr Res* 13:932-6.
10. Mertin J. Essential fatty acids and cell-mediated immunity. *Progr Lipid Res* 1981; 20:851-6.
11. Erickson K.L., Adams D.A., McNeill C.J. (1983) Dietary lipid modulation of immune responsiveness. *Lipids* 1983; 18:468-74.
12. Koletzko B., Schroten H. (1992) Ernährung und Immunfunktionen. In: Wahn U., Seeger R., Wahn V., eds. Pädiatrische Allergologie und Immunologie in Klinik und Praxis. 2. Aufl., Stuttgart: Gustav Fischer Verlag (in press).
13. Pitkänen O., Hallman M., Andersson S. Generation of free radicals in lipid emulsion used in parenteral nutrition. *Pediatr Res* 1990; 1991:56-9.
14. Kanazawa K., Ashida H., Minamoto S., Danno G., Natake M. (1988) The effect of orally administered linoleic acid and its autooxidation products on intestinal mucose in rat. *J Nutr Sci Vitaminol* 34:363-73.
15. Begin M.E. (1990) Fatty acids, lipid peroxidation and disease. *Proc Nutr Soc* 49:261-7.
16. Wispe J.R., Bell E.F., Roberts R.J. (1985) Assessment of lipid peroxidation in newborn infants and rabbits by measurements of expired ethane and pentane: influence of parenteral lipid infusion. *Pediatr Res* 19:374-9.
17. Horwitt M.K. (1974) Status of human requirements for vitamin E. *Am J Clin Nutr* 27:1182-93.
18. Bunnell R.H., de Ritter E., Rubin SH. (1975) Effect of feeding polyunsaturated fatty acids with a low vitamin E diet on blood levels of tocopherols in men performing hard labour. *Am J Clin Nutr* 28:706-11.
19. Holman R.T., Johnson S.B., Hatch T.F. (1982) A case of human linolenic acid deficiency involving neurological abnormalities. *Am J Clin Nutr* 35:617-23.
20. Bjerve K.S., Fischer S., Alme K. (1987) Alpha-linolenic acid deficiency in man: effect of ethyl linolenate on plasma and erythrocyte fatty acid composition and biosynthesis of prostanoids. *Am J Clin Nutr* 46:570-6.
21. Koletzko B. (1987) Omega-3-fatty acid requirements. *Am J Clin Nutr* 46:374.
22. Koletzko B., Cunnane S.C. (1988) Human alpha-linolenic acid deficiency. *Am J Clin Nutr* 47:1084-5.

23. Anderson G.J., Connor W.E. (1988) On the demonstration of ω-3 essential-fatty-acid deficiency in humans. *Am J Clin Nutr* 49:585-7.
24. Leyton J., Drury P.J., Crawford M.A. (1987) Differential oxidation of saturated and unsaturated fatty acids *in vivo* in the rat. *Br J Nutr* 57:383-93.
25. Koletzko B. (1992) Fats for brains. *Eur J Clin Nutr* (in press).
26. ESPGAN Committee on Nutrition (1991) Aggett PJ., Haschke F., Heine W., Hernell O., Launiala K., Rey J., Rubino A., Schöch G., Senterre J., Tormo R. Committee report. Comment on the composition of cow's milk based follow-up formulas. *Acta Paediatr Scand* 79:250-4.
27. Koletzko B., Bremer HJ. (1989) Fat content and fatty acid composition of infant formulas. *Acta Paediatr Scandiatr* 78:513-21.
28. Ballabriga A., Martinez M. (1976) Changes in erythrocyte lipid stroma in the premature infant according to dietary fat composition. *Acta Paediatr Scand* 65:705-9.
29. Putnam J.C., Carlson S.E., de Voe P., Barness LA. (1982) The effect of variations of dietary fatty acid composition on erythrocyte phosphatidylcholine and phosphatidylethanolamine in human infants. *Am J Clin Nutr* 36:106-14.
30. Carlson S.E., Rhodes P.G., Ferguson M.G. (1986) Docosahexaenoic acid status of preterm infants at birth and following feeding with human milk or formula. *Am J Clin Nutr* 44:798-804.
31. Koletzko B., Schmidt E., Bremer H.J., Haug M., Harzer G. (1989) Effects of dietary long-chain polyunsaturated fatty acids on the essential fatty acid status of premature infants. *Eur J Pediatr* 148:669-75.
32. Carlson S.E., Werkman S.H., Peeples J.M., Cooke R.J., Wilson W.M. Plasma phospholipid arachidonic acid and growth and development of preterm infants. In: Koletzko B., Okken A., Rey J., Salle B., van Biervielt JP., eds. Recent advances in infant feeding. Stuttgart: Thieme Verlag (in press).
33. Uauy R., Birch D., Birch E., Tyson J., Hoffmann D. (1990) Effect of dietary omega-3 fatty acids on retinal function of very-low-birth-weight neonates. *Pediatr Res* 28: 485-92.
34. Koletzko B., Thiel I., Abiodun P.O. (1992) The fatty acid composition of human milk in Europe and Africa. *J Pediatr* (in press).
35. Koletzko B., Thiel I., Abiodun P.O. (1991) Fatty acid composition of human milk in Nigeria. *Z Ernährungswiss J Nutr Sci* (in press).
36. Koletzko B., Mrotzek M., Bremer H.J. (1988) Fatty acid composition of mature human milk in Germany. *Am J Clin Nutr* 47:954-9.
37. Koletzko B., Müller J. (1990) Cis- and trans-isometric fatty acids in plasma lipids of newborn infants and their mothers. *Biol Neonate* 57:172-8.
38. Koletzko B., Braun M. (1991) Arachidonic acid and early human growth: is there a relation? *Ann Nutr Metab* 35:128-31.

15

Essential fatty acid requirements in premature infants

G. PUTET

Service de Néonatologie et de Réanimation Néonatale, Hôpital Debrousse, 69322 Lyon Cedex 05, France

The purpose of my presentation was to speak about essential fatty acids (EFA) requirements in premature infants. Because most of it has been already discussed since the beginning of this meeting, I am going to stress out only a few points which appear important to realize if essential fatty acids intake recommendations are to be made for very low birth weight infants.

Polyunsaturated fatty acids (PUFA) deposition in preterm and term infants

First, I would like to comment data on intrauterine accretion of EFA during the last trimester. The total amount of the n-6 fatty acids which are deposited each week during the last trimester has been estimated to be around 3 000 to 4 000 mg [1] (*Table 1*). However, it is important to realise that only 1 to 3% of this amount will be deposited in the brain. Similar remarks can be said about the n-3 family: around 470 mg are deposited per week but only 3 to 4% of this amount will be within the brain. Most of the rest of these fatty acids will be deposited in brown and white adipose tissu. From such data it is very difficult to set some kind of level for optimal intake because there are differences in data and because we do not really know up to which extend EFA deposited in adipose tissue can be utilized subsequently.

It has been shown an important difference in the total amount of the linoleic acid deposition between foetuses of different countries [2]. For instance British foetuses (*Table II*) have a lower linoleic acid increment than Dutch foetuses certainly as a result of differences in maternal diets which induce variations in human milk fatty acid

Table I. Intrauterine accretion of EFA during the last trimester of development (adapted from Clandinin [1]): most of n-6 and n-3 EFA are deposited in brown and white adipose tissue

		n-6	n-3
Brain	(mg/week)	40.9	21.8
Cerebellum	"	1.78	0.37
Spinal	"	0.095	0.014
Liver	"	13.5	3.76
Brown adipose T.	"	203	19.6
White adipose T.	"	2580	367
Others	"	817	34.1
Total/week	(mg)	3660	469
Total/day	(mg)	522	67

Table II. Increments of linoleic acid in the body fat (adapted from Southgate and Pavey, see [8]): note the difference between British and Dutch foetuses

Gestation (days)	Average total fat in body (g)	Linoleic acid increment			
		British		Dutch	
		Total fatty acids %	Gain mg/d	Total %	Gain mg/d
160	6	5.3		5.3	
180	23	4.8	38.5	5.1	38.5
200	49	4.2	48.0	4.8	59.0
220	97	3.6	71.5	4.5	101
240	165	3.0	73.5	4.2	128
260	265	2.4	70.5	3.9	171
280	476	1.8	111.0	3.7	364

composition [3]. Linoleic acid represents only 1.8% of the total fat (which means an accretion rate of around 110 mg per day) versus 3.7% (which represents around 300-400 mg pr day). So it is almost a three to four fold difference in linoleic acid deposition between these two foetuses. What is the right situation? Again, in setting a level for optimal accretion rate (and therefore optimal intake) we should consider very carefully what is the best model to look at.

Another interesting point to be discussed is the respective accretion rate of EFA and their derivatives in brain during the last trimester of pregnancy and during the first ten weeks of life in term infants [1, 4]. during the last trimester the deposition rate of n-6 FA in the brain is estimated [1] around 33 mg per week (*Table III*), most of them being not linoleic acid itself but its derivatives; if we substract linoleic and arachidonic acids from the total amount of n-6 FA deposited, we can calculate that at least one third of this total amount will be n-6 fatty acids derived from linoleic acid by desaturation and elongation process. Same calculations and commentaries can be done during the first ten weeks of the extrauterine life in term infants (*Table III*). This underlines the quantitative importance of n-6 and n-3 fatty acids which are derived from linoleic and alpha linolenic acids and deposited in brain tissue during this period of life.

Table III. Fatty acid accretion rates in infants brain and cerebellum (mg/week) (adapted from Clandinin [1, 4]): note the quantitative importance of linoleic and alpha linolenic derivatives. a: total n-6 minus linoleic acid; b: total n-6 minus linoleic arachidonic acid; c: total n-3 minus alphalinolenic acid

	Extra-uterine (0-10 wks) Term mg/wk	Intra-uterine (26-41 wks) Preterm mg/wk
Total n-6	82.4	32.83
Total n-3	5.5	14.63
Total n-9	65.5	31.21
n-6 minus 18:2(a)	79.7	32.34
n-6 minus 18:2 20:4(b)	33.2	11.95
n-3 minus 18:3(c)	6.13	14.47

PUFA and milks: adequate intakes?

It is possible to estimate the intakes of n-3 and n-6 fatty acids of infants fed human milk and an estimation of these intakes is given in *Table IV*. These figures have been calculated using published data [5, 6] on human milk composition and a milk volume intake of 180 ml/kg/day. Thus, we can calculate that the total amount of n-6 FA (which would be given to the infants at this level of milk intake) varies from 590 mg/kg/day to 800 mg/kg/day; it is important to consider that 20% of it is not linoleic acid but its derivatives. Same estimations can be made with n-3 FA with the conclusion that almost 30 to 50% of the n-3 FA intake is not alpha linolenic acid itself but its derivatives.

Therefore the preterm infant either will be given human milk and will receive these amounts of various PUFA derived from linoleic acid and alpha linolenic acids or will have to have the enzymatic capacity to elongate and desaturate linoleic and alpha linolenic acids, a situation to which he is confronted when fed cow's milk formula.

Table IV. N-6 and n-3 fatty acids intakes in infants fed human milk (180 ml/kg/d) according to human milk composition. A: mature human milk at day 29 (in [6]); B: human milk at day 15 [5]. Note the relatively important content of linoleic and alpha linolenic derivatives

	A mg/kg/d	B mg/kg/d
18:2 n-6	720.00	518.00
18:3	65.00	2.00
20:2	29.00	18.00
20:3	25.00	18.00
20:4	1.00	25.00
22:2	9.00	–
22:3	–	3.00
22:4	4.00	5.00
22:5	tr	2.00
Total n-6	852.00	591.00
Total n-6 minus 18:2 n-6	132.00	73.00
18:3 n-3	60.00	51.00
18:4	–	14.00
20:4	–	3.00
20:5	9.00	6.00
22:5	4.00	6.00
22:6	11.00	16.00
Total n-3	84.00	96.00
Total n-3 minus 18:3 n-3	24.00	45.00

In *Table V*, FA composition of different milk is given. It is clear that cow's milk has only a small amount of linoleic acid and almost none of its derivatives and no derivatives of alpha linolenic acid. Recent formulas are usually supplemented with linoleic and linolenic acids and linoleic acid content varies from 10 to 20% and linolenic acid from 1 to 2% of the total FA. Thus, the next important point to consider is the effect of adding linoleic and linolenic acid in adequate amount and with an adequate ratio between them.

In order to discuss this last point I looked at Putman's data published in 1982 (*Table VI*) [7]. In this publication Putman reported the effect of different levels of dietary essential fatty acids intakes on the fatty acid composition of erythrocyte phosphatidylcholine (PC) and phosphatidylethanolamine (PE) in human term infants. Human milk was compared with two formula: formula A and B. Formula B contained more linoleic and more alpha linolenic acids than formula A (*see Table VI*). It can be seen that:

Essential fatty acid requirements in premature infants

Table V. Fatty acids composition of human milk (HM) [6], cow's milk and preterm formula (A to F). None of the formulas quoted here contain n-6 or n-3 derivatives

	HM (ref)	Cow's milk	Preterm formula					
			A	B	C	D	E	F
C4-C10	0.9	9.1	31.7	43.1	42.6	38.6	31.8	13.5
12:0	6.7	3.6	1.6	1.4	1.3	12.2	14.9	12.7
14:0	7.8	11.8	4.7	4.5	4.9	4.7	5.8	5.4
16:0	22.5	36.6	15.9	13.5	13.8	7.5	6.8	10.1
18:0	8.0	8.1	4.3	4.05	6.4	1.7	2.3	5.1
20:0								
22:0								
24:0	0.14							
14:1	0.5	1.5	1.0	1.5				0.2
16:1	4.1	3.2	0.8	1.5	1.3	0.1	0.2	0.7
18:1	34.0	17.7	17.9	16.0	19.2	12.4	10.0	34.2
20:1	0.9	1.0				0.6	0.9	0.3
22:1								
n-6								
18:2	10.0	2.1	19.4	18.1	9.3	22.4	17.4	14.9
18:3	0.9							
20:2	0.39							
20:3	0.34							
20:4	0.39	0.4						
22:2	0.12							
22:3								
22:4	0.06							
22:5								
n-3								
18:3	0.83	1.7	0.9		1.2	0.6	0.9	2.3
18:4								
20:4								
20:5	0.13							
22:5	0.06							
22:6	0.16							

1. An increase in linoleic acid content (as realized in formula A) induced an increase in erythrocyte PC and PE linoleic acid content but not in its n-6 derivatives.

2. A further increase both in linoleic and alpha linolenic acids content (formula B) induced a further increase in PC and PE erythrocyte content of these fatty acids but not in their derivatives: furthermore the 22:5 n-6 and 22:6 n-3 (DHA) contents were decreased compared to human milk, showing the possibility of some inhibition of the desaturation process when linoleic and alphalinolenic supplementation is inadequate or n-6/n-3 ratio is unbalanced.

Table VI. Human milk, formula A, formula B, fatty acids content and fatty acid composition of term infant erythrocyte phosphatidylethanolamine (PE) and phosphatidylcholine (PC) (expressed as weight % of total acid methyl esters) in term infants fed these diets (adapted from Putman et al. [7])

Fatty acids	Human milk	PE %	PC %	Formula A	PE %	PC %	Formula B	PE %	PC %
18:2 n-6	15.8	4.9	18.2	14	7.7	22.0	45	12.6	29
20:2	0.4	0.2	0.4		0.4	0.4		0.9	0.8
20:3	0.4	1.3	2.0	tr	1.8	1.7	tr	1.6	1.2
20:4	0.6	26.5	8.4		22.3	5.3		22.2	4.6
22:4	0.2	9.7	1.2	tr	8.5	0.8	tr	9.5	0.7
22:5	0.1	1.8	0.4		1.8	0.3		1.2	0.1
18:3 n-3	0.8	0.2	0.2	1.2	0.3	0.2	5.0	0.5	0.3
20:5	0.1	0.5	0.4		0.9	0.2		0.9	0.3
22:5	0.1	3.2	0.5		2.7	0.4		3.7	0.4
22:6	0.1	6.8	1.9		3.2	0.8		3.9	0.8
%PUFA > 18C	1.9	50.5	16.7	ND	42.5	10.7	ND	44.7	9.5
%n-3 PUFA	1.1	10.7	3.1	1.2	7.4	1.6	5.0	9.1	2.0
%n-6 PUFA	17.4	44.5	31.2	14	42.3	30.6	45.1	48.1	36.1
%n-3 PUFA > 18C	0.3	10.5	2.9	ND	7.0	1.4	ND	8.5	1.7
%n-6 PUFA > 18C	1.6	39.6	12.8	ND	34.6	8.5	ND	35.5	7.3
n-6/n-3									

What is actually recommended for preterm infants

Some recommendations on linoleic and alpha linolenic acids intakes for preterm infants have been made by several committees (only those specifically designed for the premature infant have been reported):
– American Academy of Pediatrics (1985) [8]: Linoleic acid: "at least 3% of total calories".
– Canadian Paediatric Society (1981) [9]: Linoleic acid: "3% of total energy or 300 μg/100 cal".
– European Society for Paediatric Gastroenterology and Nutrition (1987) [10]: (1) Linoleic acid: "should account for at least 4-5% of total energy" (0,5 mg/100 kcal upper limit: "20% of total fatty acids (i.e. up to 1.4 g/100 kcal)"; (2) linolenic "should account for at least 0.5% of total energy (i.e. 55 mg/100 kcal)".
None of them have discussed the potential need for adequate intakes of n-6 and n-3 derivatives for the rapidly growing very low birth weight infants. Up to now there is no clinical evidence that they need them. However, as discussed during this

meeting data are coming [10, 11, 12 and see previous chapters] showing that inadequate intakes of linoleic and alphalinolenic acids or the lack of some derivatives lead to biological modifications of which long term functional consequences have not been yet fully demonstrated.

References

1. Clandinin M.T., Chapell J.E., Leong S., Heim T., Swyer P.R., Chance G.W. (1980) Intrauterine fatty acid accretion rates in human brain: implication for fatty acids requirements. *Early Hum Dev* 4(2): 121-9.
2. Widdowson E.M., Southgate D.A.T., Hey E.N. (1979) Body composition of the fetus and infant. In: Visser H.K.A., ed. *Nutrition and Metabolism of the fetus and infant.* The Hague: Martinus Nijhoff Publisher, 169-77.
3. Lammi-Keefe C.J., Jensen G. (1984) Lipids in human milk: a review. 2: composition and fat-soluble vitamins. *J Pediatr Gastroenterol Nutr* 3: 172-98.
4. Clandinin M.T., Chapell J.E., Leong S., Heim T., Swyer P.R., Chance G.W. (1980) Extrauterine fatty acid accretion rates in human brain: implication for fatty acids requirements. *Early Hum Dev* 4(2):131-8.
5. Clandinin M.T., Chappell J.E., Heim T., Swyer P.R., Chance G.W. (1981) Fatty acid utilisation in perinatal de novo synthesis of tissues. *Early Hum Dev* 5:355-66.
6. Harzer G., Haug M., Dieterich I., Gentner P.R. (1983) Changing patterns of human milk lipids in the course of the lactation and during the day. *Am J Clin Nutr* 37:612-21.
7. Putman J.C., Carlson S.E., Devoc P.W., Barness L.A. (1982) The effects of variations in dietary fatty acids on the fatty acid composition of erythrocyte phosphatidylcholine and phosphatylethanolimine in human infants. *Am J Clin Nutr* 36:106-14.
8. American Academy of Pediatrics, Committee on Nutrition. (1985) Nutritional needs of low-birth-weight infants. *Pediatrics* 75: 976-86.
9. Canadian Paediatric Society. (1981) Nutrition Committee Feeding the low-birth-weight infant. *Can Med Ass J* 124:1301-11.
10. ESPGAN (1987) Committee on nutrition of the preterm infant. Nutrition and feeding of preterm infants. *Acta Paediatr Scand* suppl. 336.
11. Delucchi L., Pita M.L., Faus M.J., Periago J.C., Gil A. (1987) Changes in the fatty acid composition of plasma and red blood cell membrane during the first hours of life in human neonate. *Early Hum Dev* 15:85-93.
12. Carlson S.E., Rhodes P.G., Ferguson M.G. (1986) Docosahexaenoic acid status of preterm infants at birth and following feeding with human milk or formula. *Am J Clin Nutr* 44:798-804.

16

Omega-3 and omega-6 fatty acid supplementation in infant formulas

G. SAWATZKI

Milupa AG, Bahnstrasse,
D-6382 Friedrichsdorf/Ts, Germany

Talking about supplementation of infant formulas as a person coming from an infant formula-producing company is a somewhat delicate task. On one hand, you know a lot of the solutions and problems, on the other hand you normally would not talk about things which are kept mostly secret in all companies. Therefore, I will give a more general short review, which will be based on the information which is already published. This will be of course more from the technical literature and especially from patents. So, in this way, I will try to show you the possibilities available and the restrictions to enrich infant formulas with polyunsaturated omega-3 and omega-6 fatty acids.

Table Ia shows the fatty acid spectrum of human milk, a conventional infant formula and a new experimental formula, which we have produced. A possible ingredient list (*Table Ib*) of the fat blend is also given, according to our patent. Today, there is no great problem to achieve an infant formula with exactly the fatty acid spectrum of human milk up to a chain length of 18 carbon atoms. Especially the desired content of linoleic and alpha-linolenic acid can be obtained by using special ingredients. Such a spectrum is already available in many infant formulas on the market and it is generally known which components you can use today to get exactly this spectrum.

But, I think the more interesting problem is how to get the C20 and C22 omega-3 and omega-6 fatty acids. Today, there is no acceptable solution available on the market and I just want to go into the problems. Why don't we have such a formula now and what are the ways to get such a formula in the future? Enriching the formulas only with fish oil will not give you the same spectrum, which you can find in human milk, because fish oils contain no arachidonic acid, or at least very, very low amounts. Therefore, you cannot reach a spectrum similar to human milk by just using fish oil. I do not want to discuss whether you have to enrich formulas or not with these polyunsaturated fatty acids, I just want to show the way how it may be performed in the future.

Essential fatty acids and infant nutrition

Table Ia. Fatty acid composition (wt %) of human milk, a commercial available formula and an experimental new formula

	Human milk	Formula	New formula
C12-0	5.5	5.2	4.7
C14-0	7.2	3.8	3.7
C16-0	23.1	28.1	28.5
C18-0	8.4	8.4	9.2
C18-1ω9	35.0	33.2	36.5
C18-2ω6	11.8	12.6	11.7
C18-3ω3	0.77	0.77	0.63
C20-3ω6	0.4	nd	0.04
C20-4ω6	0.4	nd	0.23
C22-5ω3	tr	nd	0.05
C22-6ω3	0.2	nd	0.08

Table Ib. Example of a fat blend

4.0%	liverfat (pig/cow)
2.5%	fish oil
29.0%	oleo oil
4.5%	corn oil
7.0%	soya oil
38.0%	palm oil
15.0%	coconut-/palm kernel oil

As demonstrated in *Table Ia*, it is now possible to obtain a formula with exactly this spectrum which is very similar to human milk. The content of linoleic and alpha linolenic acid is quite of the same amounts, which you can find in human milk. Moreover, you have the arachidonic acid in the amounts nearly to those you can find in human milk and also the docosahexaenoic acid. Now, we have to look to the types of fat for the blends you have to use to get exactly this spectrum. For instance, you can use liver fat (*Table II*). This might be a special problem, because getting pig's or cow's liver fat with the quality you need is not very easy. These may contain contaminants as a result of the treatment of the animals. In addition you may use a blend of fish oils, corn oil, soybean oil, palm oil and coconut/palm-kernel oil. In the following tables the different spectra for these different ingredients will be given. There is butter fat (*Table III*) which is the basis for some infant formulas. Sometimes infant formulas are produced without butter fat, because of certain problems. There might be an occurrence of trans-fatty acids, which depends on how the butter fat was produced. You have very low amounts of linoleic acid, which you should increase and sometimes you have very little arachidonic acid and eicosapentaenoic acid, as omega-6 and omega-3 fatty acids, but they are very low. If you want to increase the amount of linoleic acid by putting in some plant oils, then you face the problem that the long-chain polyunsaturated fatty acids decrease. Thus, an often used plant oil like palm oil (*Table IV*) gives especially high amounts of oleic acid. Another oil used is coconut/palm-kernel oil (*Table V*). In this oil there

Table II. Liver fat

Fatty acids		wt %
C16-0	palmitic acid	6.1
C18-0	stearic acid	23.5
C18-1ω9	oleic acid	18.2
C18-2ω6	linoleic acid	14.1
C20-2ω6	eicosadienoic acid	0.4
C20-3ω6	eicosatrienoic acid	0.6
C20-4ω6	arachidonic acid	13.9
C22-4ω6	docosatetraenoic acid	1.3
C22-5ω3	docosapentaenoic acid	1.4
C22-6ω3	docosahexaenoic acid	0.6

Table III. Butter fat

Fatty acids		wt %
C12-0	lauric acid	3.2
C14-0	myristic acid	11.9
C16-0	palmitic acid	33.9
C18-0	stearic acid	11.1
C18-1ω9	oleic acid	23.0
C18-1t	elaidic acid	2.6
C18-2ω6	linoleic acid	1.7
C20-4ω6	arachidonic acid	0.17
C20-5ω3	eicosapentaenoic acid	0.13

Table IV. Palm oil

Fatty acids		wt %
C16-0	palmitic acid	23.1
C18-0	stearic acid	4.1
C18-1ω9	oleic acid	52.0
C18-2ω6	linoleic acid	16.5
C18-3ω3	alpha-linolenic acid	0.3

are very high levels of lauric acid. Normally, we need some lauric acid but not such a high amount and therefore you have to restrict the use of this coconut/palm-kernel oil. All these oils like palm-kernel oil, coconut oil and most other commonly used plant oils face the same problem: you do not get C20 and C22 long chain polyunsaturated fatty acids. This is quite the same for soybean oil (*Table VI*), which gives you high amounts of linoleic and also alpha-linolenic acid. This oil also shows small amounts of the C20 fatty acids, but there are not any of the highly desaturated C20- and C22-fatty acids of the omega-3 and omega-6 series.

Table V. Coconut/palm-kernel oil

Fatty acids		wt %
C8-0	caprylic acid	2.7
C10-0	capric acid	3.8
C12-0	lauric acid	45.6
C14-0	myristic acid	18.5
C16-0	palmitic acid	10.3
C18-0	stearic acid	3.1
C18-1ω9	oleic acid	15.5

Table VI. Soybean oil

Fatty acids		wt %
C16-0	palmitic acid	10.3
C18-0	stearic acid	3.8
C18-1ω9	oleic acid	22.6
C18-2ω6	linoleic acid	53.9
C18-3ω3	alpha-linolenic acid	5.9
C20-1ω9	eicosenic acid	0.8
C20-2ω6	eicosadienoic acid	0.5

Table VII. Evening primrose oil

Fatty acids		wt %
C16-0	palmitic acid	6.5
C18-0	stearic acid	1.6
C18-1ω9	oleic acid	10.0
C18-2ω6	linoleic acid	72.0
C18-3ω6	gamma-linolenic acid	8.6
C18-3ω3	alpha-linolenic acid	0.3

Therefore soybean oil is an oil which does not contain considerable amounts of the highly desaturated C22 fatty acids.

Now, there are some new oils available, so far not used in infant formulas, only just experimentally. There is evening primrose oil (*Table VII*), for instance. This oil is an interesting source for the gamma-linolenic acid, and it also contains high amounts of linoleic acid. But there are not any of the C20 and the C22 fatty acids. Another oil is borage oil (*Table VIII*) which may be used, but there are not any of the C22 of the omega-6 or omega-3 fatty acids. There are considerable amounts of the C18 unsaturated fatty acids like gamma-linolenic and linoleic acid. Moreover, you have the problem with the erucic acid. Another oil is the blackcurrant kernel oil (*Table IX*) which is in the testing phase by another company, but it is not in infant formulas on the market. With this oil you may get a little more of the gamma-

Table VIII. Borage oil

Fatty acids		wt %
C16-0	palmitic acid	9.0
C18-0	stearic acid	3.0
C18-1ω9	oleic acid	13.8
C18-2ω6	linoleic acid	44.0
C18-3ω6	gamma-linolenic acid	21.2
C18-3ω3	alpha-linolenic acid	0.2
C20-1ω9	eicosenic acid	3.7
C22-1ω9	erucic acid	2.3

Table IX. Blackcurrant kernel oil*

Fatty acids		wt %
C16-0	palmitic acid	6.4
C18-0	stearic acid	1.3
C18-1ω9	oleic acid	10.3
C18-2ω6	linoleic acid	46.5
C18-3ω6	gamma-linolenic acid	18.2
C18-3ω3	alpha-linolenic acid	13.6
C18-4ω3	octadecatetraenoic acid	3.7

* Traitler H., Wille H.J., Studer A. (1986) Fraktionierung mehrfach ungesättigter Fettsäuren aus verschiedenen natürlichen Rohstoffen. *Fat-Science-Technology* 88: 378-82.

linolenic acid and alpha-linolenic acid, but you don't get the C20 and C22 fatty acids with this source.

Now, let us have a look at the fish oils (*Table X*) like cod liver oils, which have very little arachidonic acid, but relatively high amounts of w3 long-chain fatty acids like eicosapentaenoic acid and docosahexaenoic acid. For all fish oils you have the problem, that you do not have enough of arachidonic acid.

Therefore, it can be summarized that there are only a few sources for arachidonic acid. The only ones now available on the market are these liver oils or liver fats from animals, but leaving us with many problems of contaminants. Then you will get enough of arachidonic acid. This might be a source for arachidonic acid, if you want to make an infant formula containing arachidonic acid, containing the same amounts of these fatty acids which you will find normally in human milk. In contrast to the use of fish oil, you will avoid too much of docosahexaenoic acid and the eicosapentaenoic acid, but because of the problems, this is not an acceptable solution. What will the future bring? The future may be fungal oils or single cell oils (*Table XI*) and this is something which you face, if you are doing research in the industry. Many patents of Japanese origin are available about these fungal oils and they are very high in arachidonic acid.

They also contain gamma-linolenic acid, but they are especially very interesting as sources for arachidonic acid. What is the problem with fungal oils? Mortierella

Table X. Cod liver oil

Fatty acids		wt %
C14-0	myristic acid	3.6
C16-0	palmitic acid	10.2
C16-1	palmitoleic acid	9.2
C18-0	stearic acid	2.9
C18-1ω9	oleic acid	23.3
C18-2ω6	linoleic acid	2.0
C18-3ω3	alpha-linolenic acid	11.5
C20-2ω6	eicosadienoic acid	2.3
C20-4ω6	arachidonic acid	0.5
C20-5ω3	eicosapentaenoic acid	9.8
C22-1ω11	cetoleic acid	8.2
C22-5ω3	docosapentaenoic acid	1.2
C22-6ω3	docosahexaenoic acid	11.5

Table XI. Fungal oil. Organism: *Mortierella elongata (Phycomycetes)**

Fatty acids		wt %
C16-0	palmitic acid	9.4
C18-0	stearic acid	3.5
C18-1ω9	oleic acid	50.9
C18-2ω6	linoleic acid	8.2
C18-3ω6	gamma-linolenic acid	3.5
C20-4ω6	arachidonic acid	16.5

* Yamada H., Shimizu S., Shinmen Y., Kawashima H., Akimoto K.. (1988) Production of arachidonic acid and eicosapentaenoic acid by microorganisms. In: Applewhite T.H., ed. Proceedings of the World Conference on Biotechnology for the Fats and Oils Industry, Glenview, USA: Am. Oil Chemist's Society Kraft Inc.: 173-7.

is sometimes known as a pathogen for human beings and you cannot use it without making all the toxicological evaluations, which you have to do as a careful infant formula producer. You may grow these cells in big fermentors and you can make a lot of these fungal oils, but the extraction processes for these fungal oils are not available on the market and you have to develop new processes. These are a lot of very special aspects, just to show the problems you have in making infant formulas just with a fatty acid spectrum like that of human milk. Today, you cannot get these raw materials suitable for infant formulas.

Another problem is directly connected with the use of the long chain polyunsaturated fatty acids: you are confronted with the problems of oxidative damage during processing. This is a severe problem, because there might be no benefit of putting in all these polyunsaturated fatty acids, when they are oxidized during the process. This is very important, especially when you want to have a long term stable infant formula. Then you have to get rid of this problem of oxidation.

The second problem is that if you are using fish oils, which is one possible source for these polyunsaturated fatty acids, this formula will not be used by the mother, because it stinks like fish. That is a very practical problem and there are only very few fish oils on the market which have been desodorised. Desodorising of the fish oil brings a new problem: you are using high temperatures and special ingredients and then you are facing the problem of getting trans fatty acids.

These are most of the practical problems and today we have no possibility to get a real stable infant formula, which is exactly showing the spectrum of fatty acids which you can find in human milk. We have to work very hard during the next few years, maybe five years, to really find solutions for all these problems which I presented.

SESSION VII

General discussion

Chairman: Jean REY (France)

General discussion

Chairman: We shall start the discussion but we will try to organize the discussion and discuss many points and the main point is the human milk model. Perhaps we can return to the morning session of yesterday for a moment, on the fundamental aspect of the metabolism of the elongation and desaturation of the precursor. When some of you propose to mimic human milk and to add long chain fatty acid, at least for term infant, I believe that you suppose there is no delta-6 or delta-5 or delta-4-desaturase activity. If you think that there is some desaturase activity, you can propose that the precursor is in sufficient quantity and can provide enough long chain polyunsaturated fatty acids. So in the audience can somebody try to make a short statement on the delta-6-desaturase activity, is it enough or not enough in term infant or preterm infant?

G. Béréziat: Two years ago we published preliminary works in the neonate on delta-5 or delta-6-desaturase activity. In the late stage of gestation, in humans, there is a great increase in delta-5-desaturase activity. But I wonder if there is any sufficient delta-6-desaturase activity at birth.

J.M. Bourre: Considering the delta-6-desaturase activity, it is higher in the young or even in the foetus, but it does not mean that this activity is sufficient to face all the very long chains which are needed. The other point is that these long chain fatty acids being present in the human milk during the evolution from the ape to the human must be used for something. For the moment we don't know why, we don't know how, but they are present and they have some role. We have to remain modest. We know that they are present and we have to add them. So coming back to the delta-6-desaturase, the last speaker mentioned the usefulness of various oils as evening primrose oil or blackcurrant oil, for instance and for the moment there is absolutely no reason to add these oils as providing gammalinolenic acid. The only base to add these kinds of oils is reduced delta-6-desaturase activity, which is precisely not the case in the young. There is absolutely no reason at any time, even during ageing to add these oils. A short comment on using fish oil. We have to be very, very careful because those fish oils on the market have a high amount of eicosapentanoic acid which means reduced amount of cervonic acid. We have to find some fish mutants providing higher amount of cervonic acid and lower amount of EPA. We have also to take into account that those fish oils do give large amounts, more than 50% of the very long chain fatty acids and the metabolism of those fatty acids is totally ignored for the moment.

Chairman: Can we stay on your first point, you are very finalist and I agree with this philosophy, but are we sure that these long chain fatty acids are not an obligatory component of the cell membrane, of the membrane of the fat globule, can somebody answer this question?

M. Hamosh: What we really don't know exactly is the amount of very long chain polyunsaturate fatty acids which are present in milk globule membrane. I think we have a lot of work to do, and I think we should look particularly at the preterm and the term milk, the whole idea of prematurity is 20 years old. All the full term infants are probably doing all right.

I don't think there is a huge difference in IQ between people who have been breast fed and people who have been bottle fed! So I really think we have to think about the premature infants; what does the premature get, how does the mammary gland function in preterm and full term? Maybe we should put the emphasis on having more premature infants fed human milk rather than formula, and maybe put the emphasis into either collecting it, trying to maintain the function in a mother delivering prematurely, or banking it.

J.M. Bourre: The problem is what about brain fatty acids, and the type of fatty acids which are found in the body fat. For the moment the only data as far as I know which are available in human are Clandinin data, showing that in the newborn at term, there is sufficient amount of polyunsaturated fatty acids in the body fat in order to provide enough polyunsaturated fatty acids to the rest of the organism, in terms of alphalinolenic acid for instance, when a newborn is totally deprived in his diet in alphalinolenic acid.

Considering the fat metabolism the turnover for some fatty acids in adipose tissue is about one year. Even when there is a sufficient amount of reserves in the fat, in terms of polyunsaturated fatty acids, for the rest of the body, it's not totally clear if those reserves are useful for the rest of the body. Another point is that the phospholipids containing those very long chain fatty acids are obliged part of the globule in the milk, so they are not in fact useful. They are just structural components. However we have data showing that, in fact, more than two thirds of the polyunsaturated fatty acids with very long chain were found in the triglycerides. In this case the argument is not valuable. It has been discussed about minor components such as cerebrosides, sulfatides, gangliosides and these molecules could be speculated as being structural for sphingomyeline but certainly not for cerebrosides or sulfatides and probably not for gangliosides. These sphingolipids are providing saturated and monounsaturated fatty acids such as lignoceric acid and nervonic acid which are found in fact in the brain, so one can raise the question also what about the usefulness of some part of the milk so as to provide saturated and monounsaturated non essential fatty acid for all the tissues, including for the brain?

M. Hamosh: I would like to take up on your very interesting comments. I don't think that anything that is in the membrane is of no use, because I think that the phospholipids and the cholesterol esters are broken down and the fatty acids are of benefit to the infant. I just don't think this is just there and is destroyed.

Chairman: Sheila, yesterday you tried to prove that precursor of the n–3 series are sufficient for the metabolism of the baby and Susan was probably of a different opinion. Can you return to this point because I want to say to Jean-Marie Bourre I agree that long chain fatty acids are necessary, but necessary per se or necessary as a metabolite, as a precursor, that's a question.

General discussion

S. Innis: My studies are in piglets which, I think, are probably one of the most useful models. I think in these discussions what is very important is that we delineate between term and preterm infants, and I think the requirements of preterm infant are quite different from those of the term infant, based on our knowledge on the reserves at birth and very rapid growth.

We need to take lessons from the protein content of human milk and its inadequacies well known now for the preterm infant. I think that modelling a formula on the absolute quantity of 18:2, 18:3 contained in human milk may be inadequate for preterm infants; their requirements for 18:2, 18:3 could be a little bit higher.

Chairman: Thank you. Susan, will you comment on this?

S. Carlson: I think what I would like to say is that I do think Sheila's data in the pigs very interesting. I take some message from that because the pig's brain development is similar to the human infant. It's very interesting to me that the docosahexaenoic acid in the brain of these piglets is increasing in the animals that receive their mother's milk which has docosahexaenoic acid, and it's not increasing in the piglets which are receiving the formula. I also think it's interesting that the arachidonic acid does not seem to be affected by those formulas which do not contain arachidonic acid.

I think it's clear to me and someone else showed data earlier that arachidonic acid in human milk is incorporated into membranes of infants. Human milk fed infants tend to have higher, statistically, amounts of arachidonic acid than formula fed infants. The arachidonic acid content of the membranes is also dependent on long chain n–3 fatty acid intake. So I think it's very difficult to define an ideal supplement for babies.

When we look at babies fed human milk compared to formulas the two fatty acids that come out significantly are arachidonic acid and the docosahexaenoic acid. I think that these babies don't have tremendous problems with other desaturated fatty acids but I'm not sure of that. The question is, are they making or not the amounts that they need for normal brain development?

Chairman: Thank you very much. Dr Koletzko?

B. Koletzko: Another part of this question is, does diet matter for these infants? We noted in your data a depletion in plasma of long chain polyunsaturated, omega-6, omega-3 fatty acids, in the term infant in the first few weeks of life, in formula fed infants. Plasma phospholipids are exchanged with structural lipids. Data by in term infants, as far as I recall, show clearly that there is a close correlation between LCP long chain of brain lipids and liver lipids and I think that we can assume that plasma phospholipid composition is mostly dependent on other metabolisms which would reflect what's happening in the liver. What I really would like to know is what is the composition of the brain. I think we have to be careful about looking at a function and stating that well breast fed infants are OK.

The other problem where I think there are other indications of imbalances is for example in eicosanoid metabolism. There is a study which shows that giving as little as 100 mg of arachidonic acid per kg per day (which is about twice the amount in breast fed infants) very significantly increased prostaglandin excretion.

Chairman: Have we any information on the plasma or erythrocyte phospholipid arachidonic levels in relation to the intake of gammalinolenic or dihomogammalinolenic?
Has somebody any information on this? The question is: is supplementation with gammalinolenic sufficient to provide normal value for arachidonic or not?

C. Galli: I think there have been a few studies in the literature showing that. If you supplement the diet with dihomogammalinolenic acid or with gammalinolenic acid, actually the arachidonic acid content is not modified. The only thing which varies is the dihomogammalinolenic which accumulates.

Chairman: We discussed this morning and yesterday of data from US and Germany, on human milk and phospholipids, but we know that there is very large difference between population in the intake of linoleic acid or fish oil. Have we some information on long chain fatty acids in groups as Eskimos or in Bedouins?

J.M. Bourre: I would like to remind you that Eskimos die when they are around 50 because of brain hemorrhage, so they have no cardio-vascular diseases. Anyway it was reported, two years ago, that in fact EPA in the Eskimo human milk is only slightly increased, but not so much as the amounts which are found in the blood.

Chairman: But you have no information in infants?

J.M. Bourre: No, it was only in the milk.

M. Hamosh: This is very interesting because it's quite contrary to the data reported a few years ago by Harris, in which when you supplement the mum with high amounts of fish oil the milk reflects this increase almost immediately. The increment in the milk is directly proportional to the increment in the diet. This was an accute study done over a short period of time. I wonder whether the Eskimos through their evolution developed a certain steady mechanism in which only very little of the fish oil filters into the milk or other mechanisms, I think the discrepancy is very interesting.

C. Galli: I would like to say that eating fish oil and eating fish is quite different.

S. Innis: We studied breast milk collected from Inuit women who were eating a very traditional diet in which protein sources were largely from animal flesh and the only source for the diet oil was from marine mammals. The levels of DHA in those milks were very similar to those recorded with fish oils.

J.M. Bourre: So the other point concerning these Eskimos is that they are fed with marine mammals and the distribution of the polyunsatured fatty acids on the triglycerides are not the same in fish and in marine mammals. So what about the lipolysis of these triglycerides, this is another problem.

General discussion

M. Hamosh: The marine mammals is one big group but it turns out that, when you divide them into the different sub-groups, there are those who feed the babies once a day and those who feed them once a week. Those who feed once a day for only 1 week and those are the ones with a 50% fat in milk. I would be very interested to look at the digestion and absorption of these long chain fatty acids in these two situations.
Again we have to learn a lot but I think we have a very different species in which adipose tissue has to be deposited very fast. I don't know about the IQ of my mammals and I don't know anything about their visual acuity but this might be an interesting model.

J. Ghisolfi: I admit that fatty acid composition of human milk is very important, but what is the best human milk? Is it the milk from Eskimo woman, vegetarian woman or Arabian woman?

S. Carlson: Last year, Mr Crawford said that he didn't think we were giving enough DHA in human milk in the US. So perhaps 0,4 or 0,5% would be better than 0,1 or 0,2.

D. Hull: Just a bit of data: we did study dietary intake of Asian women who were living in London and they get very little of the longer polyunsaturated fatty acids in their diet. But they've got plenty in their circulation. There's no doubt the mother elongated. So we looked at the cord blood: there was plenty of 22:4 and 22:6. We haven't actually analysed the mother's milk. I imagine, if the mother's milk takes up the fatty acid from the mother's circulation, there are plenty of 22:6 and 20:4 in the milk of these mothers. I wonder if the Eskimo women don't take it, the other way is that they have a dietary process that makes sure that their circulation lipids have got a balance so that their milk doesn't have excesses of the more unusual long chain fatty acids.

Chairman: David, do you believe that it's the same for the two families for n–3 or n–6, because we had information that there is no correlation between arachidonic (for example) in the milk and linoleic acid in the diet, but there is some relation for the n–3 family. Perhaps it's different for the two families?

D. Hull: I wasn't making that point. I was saying that if the mother is fed a diet which is high in 18:2 and 18:3, she processes so that she got high circulating levels of the longer polyunsaturated fatty acids. The baby gets those *in utero* judged by the umbilical arterial levels of those fatty acids and I presume that the milk got plenty of those unsaturated fatty acids.

J.M. Bourre: I remember this communication: in fact although these mothers got huge amount of alphalinolenic acid in the diet the children, when being breast fed, had a deficiency in DHA in the blood and in the red blood cells, which was an argument to say that DHA could be essential to a certain extent during the development. Is that right?

S. Carlson: I'd like to tell you some data that we have on these babies that we are studying. At nine months they go on a cow's milk formula. What we are finding is that between that 9 months blood sample and 12 months blood sample, their plasma arachidonic acid levels have doubled and their linolenic acid levels go to half but there is no effect whatsoever on docosahexaenoic acid level. I don't know why. I wonder if the reason why there is no association between linolenic acid and arachidonic acid in the milk is that we are already 10% too high and that we have already overridden whatever control there may have been. Perhaps if women assumed only 2% fat from linoleic acid, their plasma would give a higher amount of arachidonic acid.

Chairman: But the baby eats meat at that time, would it be possible that arachidonic acid comes from meat?

S. Carlson: Well, I don't think it can account for going from 10 to 20% of arachidonic acid.

Chairman: Well, we had many, many data on infants, young infants during these two days but nobody has presented long chain fatty acid status in a one year old infant, for example, in relation to the diet in the first weeks of life. Have you any information on this? No.
Another question, Susan has shown this morning that visual acuity is decreased in some situations, but can we have more information on the predictive value of this visual defect. Can it be corrected with time or not?

S. Carlson: We have analysed the data for 6 months; we have done babies that have reached the year but we are waiting until we get a large enough number to do our analysis. The difference we're seeing, it's not a deficit in the controls. I wanted to emphasize that: what we're seeing is an improvement over apparent norms in the supplemented babies.

Chairman: Yes, Claudio...

C. Galli: I would like to make two comments. One: it has been emphasized mainly the importance of the fatty acids for the brain but we don't have to forget that these fatty acids are important for other systems as well. Another question I would ask the people today. Obviously the human milk has very high quantities of long chain polyunsaturates, do we know about the mechanism for the protection from oxidation in human milk? Is there any specific thing which is missing when we prepare formulas?

Chairman: Another comment, another question, someone will ask something...

G. Béréziat: As you know there are different pools in the phospholipids in red blood cells and it has been proved now that for the synthesis of eicosanoids, some pools are important, some others are not. Maybe some pools are only specialised in the

General discussion

storage of arachidonic acid and other pools in the liberation of arachidonic acid. My question is: why don't we measure the fatty acid content into the subclasses of phosphatidylcholine and phosphatidylethanolamine?

Chairman: It's expensive.

M. Hamosh: That's what I wanted to say. This is especially for the Milupa Company, if anyone funds us, we would do it.

J. Ghisolfi: I think there is another important question: what is the maximum of linoleic acid intake which is dangerous for essential fatty acid metabolism in infants?

Chairman: Susan said a few minutes ago that she believes that 10% is the maximum or 15%.

S. Carlson: I don't think it's a maximum, I'm just saying that I think that at 10% perhaps you're maybe already over a level where you're going to see a relationship between linoleic and arachidonic.

Chairman: So it's 5% of energy.

S. Carlson: The only thing that I'm aware of is that babies on very high linolenic acid intake have much lower levels of HDL cholesterols as well as LDL cholesterols. But I don't know the significance of that.

Chairman: So we have a lot of work to do for the future and we arrive at the end of this workshop. I will thank you everybody for the participation to the discussion. I will thank again Jacques Ghisolfi and Guy Putet for the organizing of the programme, a very good programme. I would like to thank also J.L. Ramet from the Milupa Company in Paris who has provided funds and friendship for this meeting.

LOUIS-JEAN
avenue d'Embrun, 05003 GAP cedex
Tél. : 92.53.17.00
Dépot légal : 712 — Octobre 1992
Imprimé en France